Microcirculation

In the same series

- Fish oil and blood-vessel wall interactions
  P. M. Vanhoutte, Ph. Douste-Blazy

- Return circulation and norepinephrine : an update
  P. M. Vanhoutte

The papers of this book were reprinted from acts of two conferences held in Cairo and in Grenada and published by John Libbey Eurotext, by authorization of the authors and the editors.

Microcirculation

Editor

M.R. Boisseau

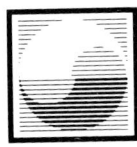

Pierre Fabre

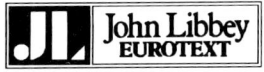

British Library Cataloguing in Publication Data
Boisseau, M.R.
 Microcirculation.
 I. Title.

ISBN 0 86 196 346 6

Editions John Libbey Eurotext
6, rue Blanche, 92120 Montrouge, France.
Tél. : (1) 47.35.85.52 – Fax : (1) 46.57.10.09

John Libbey and Company Ltd
13, Smith Yard, Summerley Street, London SW18 4HR, England
Tél. : (81) 947.27.77

John Libbey CIC
Via L. Spallanzani, 11
00161 Rome, Italy
Tél. : (06) 862.289

© 1992, Paris

Il est interdit de reproduire intégralement ou partiellement le présent ouvrage – Loi du 11 mars 1957 – sans autorisation de l'éditeur ou du Centre français du Copyright, 6 *bis*, rue Gabriel Laumain, 75010 Paris, France.

Contents

Preface
M.R. Boisseau VII

1. **Microcirculation and microrheology**
   M. R. Boisseau 1

2. **Ω-3 fatty acids and microcirculation**
   G. Bruckner 21

3. **Effect of chronic exposure to cod liver oil and Ω-3 unsaturated fatty acids on endothelium-dependent relaxations**
   C. Boulanger, V.B. Schini, H. Shimokawa, Th. F. Lüscher, P.M. Vanhoutte 31

4. **Interaction between Ω-3 fatty acid and platelet phospholipids**
   M. Lagarde, M. Groset, M. Hajarine 41

5. **Pharmacological modulation of venular permeability with some antiinflammatory drugs**
   E. Svensjö 47

6. **Hemorheological concepts in venous insufficiency and implications for treatment with *Ruscus* extract**
   C. Le Devehat, T. Khodabandehlou, M. Vimeux, G. Bondoux 57

7. **Effect of *Ruscus* extract on the capillary filtration rate**
   G. Rudofsky 69

8. **Microcirculatory responses to *Ruscus* extract in the hamster cheek pouch**
   E. Bouskela 75

Author index 87

Preface

There are many facets to the microcirculation. It can be observed directly *in vivo* as well as histologically, where its functions, especially those relating to exchanges with tissue, can be explored. This diversity of approaches has perhaps let us lose sight of its overall role. Indeed, work on spastic and vasomotor properties of microvessels, which have a direct impact on peripheral resistance, has tended to eclipse the other functions of the microcirculation. Nevertheless, the great strides in investigative methods in recent years have brought much new information on the system, most notably with respect to the role of endothelial cells.

1 – Current status of the microcirculation

The idea of a microcirculatory unit initially proposed by Merlen is now well recognized. The microvessels operate as a system of organs with their own specific functions (perfusion, exchanges, transit) and intrinsic cellular activities (e.g. endothelial cells), which should be viewed as an autonomous regulated parenchyma. The microcirculation can be conceptualized not only as a network, but also as myriad zones of activity, which both regulate and are regulated. These zones correspond to active vascular surfaces, which may be quite extensive, especially in muscle bulks. A disorder in a particular zone subserving some specific function can thus have significant pathological consequences.

An intriguing facet of the microcirculation that has emerged recently is the role of endothelial cells. Somewhat overlooked in the past, endothelial cells are now being found to have crucial and seemingly contradictory activities. Their essentially anticoagulant properties are replaced during tissue injury by a clot promoting action. They may repel or attract circulating cells, either activating them or not via production of agonists or cytokines. In addition, cellular contraction by altering the gaps between these cells modulates their permeability. The importance of this tissue can be judged by the variety of functions it performs.

The microcirculatory unit has four principle functions : vasopression (peripheral resistance), tissue exchange, permeability and cell transit (leucocytes). Endothelial cells are the essential regulators of cell transit and permeability, and participate in vasomotor control. This activity of microvessels depends, however, on the conditions of perfusion and motor pressure within the vascular lumen. Not all microcirculatory units will be open at one and the same time, and they are particularly sensitive to perfusion conditions in systemic vessels. Thus hyperpressure in the lower limbs has a marked feedback effect on the microvessels. In contrast, ischemia stops the microcirculatory flow, disrupting the delicate balance of regulating factors responding to stress and gas pressures (pO_2 and pCO_2). This can induce profound alterations in endothelial cells, and compromise attempts at reperfusion.

2 – Microcirculation and pharmacology

The microcirculation represents a good target for therapeutic intervention. This avenue is being actively explored in animal systems and in man, as well as on endothelial cells in culture. Drug action is aimed essentially at the vasomotor and permeability regulating functions of these cells since both influence peripheral and systemic pressure, as well as tissue exchanges of water and molecules.

An animal model of the microcirculation is described in the chapter by Svensjo. Fluid tends to leak between gaps in endothelial cells of the post-capillary venules, and the cells can modulate this flow of fluid by altering these gaps. Numerous agonists of this property, which act directly on endothelial cells, have been developed, while leakage is observed by the movement of fluorescent dyes. This model can be used to screen for agents with capillary sealing activity, inhibiting fluid leakage either via an immediate or a delayed action (genic action).

3 – Microcirculation and omega 3 polyunsaturates

Using quantified capillaroscopy and laser-Doppler imaging, Bruckner has investigated the influence of diets rich in polyunsaturated fatty acids on capillary blood flow in both normal and hyperlipidemic individuals. Diets rich in omega 3 polyunsaturates were found to increase flow, but only in the presence of antioxidants (vitamin E). There was no effect on systemic pressure or viscosity. A seductive suggestion is that oils rich in these fatty acids favor production of vasodilator eicosanoids on the surface of endothelial cells. These eicosanoids are highly sensitive to oxidation, and so their effects are prolonged in the presence of antioxidants.

Boulanger *et al.* report interesting results on the effects of eicosapentaenoic acid (EPA) on the production of endothelium relaxing substances from endothelial cells. EDFR/NO does not seem to be involved, although factors appear after activation by ADP. Furthermore, EPA was found to overregulate NO receptors on endothelial cells enhancing their permeability. The beneficial effect of EPA thus potentiates the action of NO. These findings corroborate results obtained on endothelial cells of pigs receiving a diet enriched in omega 3 polyunsaturates.

The effects of other polyunsaturated fatty acids are reported by Lagarde *et al.* who found a beneficial action of decosahexaenoic acid (DHA). This fatty acid accumulates in membrane phospholipids of endothelial cells and platelets, particularly in the phosphatidylethanolamine fraction, where it appears to neutralize thromboxane A2 receptors.

Omega 3 polyunsaturates and fish oils thus have an impact on both the spasticity and permeability of the microcirculation.

4 – Ruscus and microcirculation

Another interesting pharmacological application is represented by the effects of flavanoids from *Ruscus aculeatus* (water/alcoholic extract of roots) on microvessels.

Bouskela has investigated the effects of preparations of Ruscus on the hamster after oral and intravenous administration as well as by direct application. In both the systemic circulation and the microcirculation, he observed a constrictive action on a third of the veins, and a vasodilator action on a third of the arteries. The affected venules ranged in diameter from 30 m to 40 m, i.e. the post-capillary venules that are well supplied with muscle fibers. Ruscus appears to act on a-adrenergic receptors. No effects were observed on arterial pressure, and there was only a slight effect on vein collaterals. Interestingly a heat dependence was noted, with a reversal of effect at low temperatures.

Support for these findings from direct measurements on venules was obtained by Rudofsky by plethysmographic measurements of leg volume after compression on two groups of normal subjects and a group of women with chronic superficial venous insufficiency. Ruscus was found to reduce the filtration rate and the venous capacity, although it did not improve vein tone or lymphatic drainage.

In a rheological context, Le Dévéhat showed that Ruscus significantly reduced plasma viscosity, hematocrit and red cell aggregability with respect to placebo-treated controls. These actions were found to be sensitized by venous compression prior to blood sampling. The results are indicative of blockade of chronic vascular leakage, which had reduced plasma volume in these patients thereby exacerbating any rheological abnormalities. Possible mechanisms of action of Ruscus are on permeability (reduced) and venous resistance (increased) along with an interstitial anti-edema action.

These interesting findings on the local and systemic actions of such substances are perhaps not fully appreciated at the present time. It is astonishing that rheological effects of such substances can be observed on venous blood sampled from the forearm. They appear to improve perfusion and drainage of microvessels leading to a fall in pressure and hence a reduction in fluid leakage.

In general, the most useful pharmacological actions on the microcirculation are on drainage. Drugs designed to prevent accumulation of blood within venules are of particular interest as this action will also have an impact on circulating cells, especially leucocytes.

From a pathophysiological viewpoint, the role of the microcirculatory surface and the various contributions of the different parts of the network, including cardiac, digestive, muscular or cutaneous components, will be increasingly elucidated and appreciated with the advent of new investigative techniques.

In addition, microvessels represent a potential target of drug action since they lie upstream of venous thromboses, and are highly represented in ischemic zones.

Pharmacologically, fish oils and derivatives especially eicosapentaenoic acid have aroused much interest as they counteract dietary risk factors, and appear to have a direct influence on thrombotic processes involving platelets and endothelial cells.

The reader will find in the following pages much stimulating material on these exciting new approaches to the microcirculation.

M.R. Boisseau

1

Microcirculation and microrheology

M.R. Boisseau

INSERM U8, Université de Bordeaux II, 33604 Pessac, France.

Introduction

Over the past decade, increasing attention has been paid to the role of the microcirculation in the pathophysiology of a number of conditions. A microcirculation has been identified anatomically in all major organs, and its physiological role has been investigated in various animal or experimental models. Despite the paucity of studies in humans, a considerable body of knowledge has now been accumulated which has formed the subject of numerous publications and reviews of which those of Tsuchiya [77], Messmer [48], Larcan [39], Mortillaro [50], Manabe [44], Wiedeman *et al.* [85] deserve mention. Over the same period, fundamental studies on blood flow in microvessels have been carried out, especially with respect to the movement of blood cells. This has given rise to the concept of microrheology. Even more recently, the role played by endothelial cells in microrheology via cell-cell interactions has become apparent.

A number of lines of evidence point to an intimate link between microrheological phenomena and the microcirculation. Although the microcirculation is under neuro-hormonal regulation and vasomotor control, both passive and active rheological processes occur essentially in the microcirculation, as they only become significant in vessels subjected to low propulsive forces. Such processes tend to be amplified under various pathological conditions. Considerable impairment of the microcirculation may occur in vascular disease, for example, and rheological disorders need to be taken into account when evaluating the patient's condition [9]. In fact, treatment strategies aimed specifically at disorders of blood cell rheology are under development.

This chapter will outline first the histological, physiological and pathophysiological aspects of the microvessels.

The microcirculation

Microvessels

Microvessels can be considered to include all vessels with a diameter or 100 µm or less. These vessels constitute the true capillary bed, the principle site of exchanges between blood and tissues. In fact, there is no clear-cut distinction between the systemic and the microcirculation, but vessels whose diameters are of a similar order of magnitude to the those of blood cells are subjected to different hemodynamic influences, and are much more sensitive to rheological factors. They constitute a considerable reservoir of blood especially on the venous side. On the arterial side, they represent a principle source of peripheral resistance which is regulated by the sympathetic branch of the autonomic nervous system.

The microvessels encompass a large surface area, and in man, the endothelial cells lining these vessels have been estimated to weigh 3 kg. The importance of the endothelial organ which is in constant contact with blood is highlighted by recently identified actions of this tissue on both blood and muscle cells in vessels walls.

Microcirculation as an entity

There are considerable differences in the functional arrangements of microvessels, especially in parenchymatous organs (see review by Wiedeman et al. [85]). A common functional unit can, however, be identified, typified by the microcirculation in muscles, which represents the largest area of microvessels in the organism. In France, the notion of the microcirculation unit has been extensively studied by Merlen (1912-1986).

Table I shows the constitution of the microcirculation unit in the vascular tree. It consists of five principle vessel types : arterioles (100 to 40 µ) surrounded by richly innervated smooth muscle cells : pre-capillary arterioles

Table 1. Position of microvessels in the circulatory system. *Diameter* : cm for macrovessels, then µ for microvessels. *Output* : expressed as velocity of red cells in cm per sec.

Microvessels position

Vessel	Diameter (cm then µ)	Muscle	Nerves	Output (cm/sec)
Aorta (arch)	2 to 3			60
Aorta	1 to 2			30
Arterioles	100 to 40	CML^{+++}	$Symp+++$	0.5
Pre-capill. art.	30	CML^+	0	0.5
Capillaries	10 to 5 (50 % 4.5	O	0	0.005
Post-capill. venulae	20 to 30	0	0	0.01
Venules	40 to 100	CML^+	$Symp^+$	0.2 to 0.5
Veins	0.5 to 1			15 to 20
Vena cava	3			10 to 15

(30 to 40 µ) or pre-capillary sphincters associated with smooth muscle cells which are not, however, innervated (Wiedeman, 1981); true capillaries (10 to 5 µ, 50 %< 4.5 µ) with a less elaborate structure; post-capillary venules (20 to 30 µ) surrounded by pericytes with few smooth muscle cells, venules (40 to 100 µ) with few parietal smooth muscle cells and little innervation. A fundamental feature of the microvessels is their low rate of blood flow compared to systemic vessels. The lowest flow rates are found in the post-capillary venules, producing the lowest shear forces in the whole vascular tree.

The various components of the microcirculation unit have specialized functions *(Table II)*, which confer a certain functional coherence to the system. The well-innervated terminal arterioles represent the organ of perfusion of

Table 2. The «microcirculatory unit» (JF Merlen). Functional specific role for each group of microvessels.

Microcirculatory unit

100	▶ 50 à 30 µ	Arterioles Pre-capillaries arterioles	Tissue perfusion Systemic blood pressure
	10 to 5 µ	Capillaries	Interstitial tissue exchange (gas and liquids)
	20 to 30 µ	Post-capillaries venulae	Cell transit to tissues (blood cells thoroughfare)
100	◀ 40 µ	Venulae	Venous blood reservoir Venous pressure

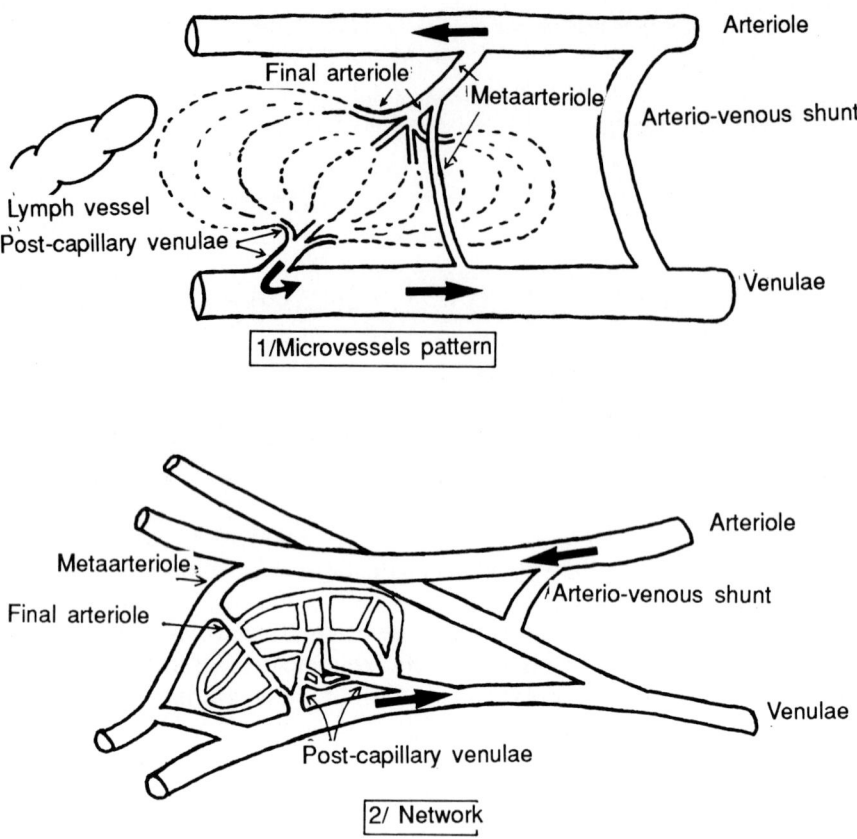

Figure 1. Schematic draft of the microcirculation. Adaptability of the network. Aspects related to microvessels of skeletal muscles.

the unit, and are the main source of peripheral resistance which is a significant regulator of blood pressure. Metabolic and mechanical regulation of the unit take place in the precapillary arterioles which adjust to alterations in arteriolar perfusion. Interstitial exchanges occur essentially in the capillaries, although water and some molecules also exchange with tissues in the venules. The postcapillary venules are an important site of cellular exchanges, and the main point of entry of leucocytes into tissues. Finally, the venules have a capacitance function in the blood reservoir. The exchange of water and small molecules between the venules and tissues can lead to a build up of venous pressure in some circumstances (orthostatic venous hyperpressure for example).

It can thus be seen there is a relationship between structure and function of the various components of the microcirculation unit. Although there are differences in the arrangement of these components in the various organs, their functions are invariably in the above-mentioned sequence.

Anatomy and Histology

The first anatomical and histological descriptions of the blood vessels go back to Harvey (1578-1657) and Malpighi (1628-1694). In recent years, the structures of microvessels have been described in detail for the various organs of the body [39, 44, 77, 85]. Without entering into details, a few essential points are worth mentioning here.
The innervation of arterioles stops at the terminal arterioles, but is extended by extra-vascular fibers.
The true capillaries have a simple mono-cellular architecture whose structure varies from organ to organ. It is fenestrated in parenchyma, discontinuous in hematopoietic organs, but continuous in skin, skeletal muscles and the nervous system.
An important anatomical feature is the presence of arteriovenous anastomoses whose shunting action is central to microcirculatory function. These anastomoses form a linked network with considerable adaptive properties. *Figure 1* shows a typical network in skeletal muscle.

Regulation of the microcirculation

Three main parameters can be regulated in the microcirculation unit. *Blood flow* is influenced by both local and general control systems. *Exchanges* with interstitial tissue and lymphatics, and *cell transit* involving rheological processes are all subjected to a number of controlling influences.

Regulation of flow and pressure

General factors

The neurohormonal regulation (baroreflexes) is coordinated by bareoreceptors situated in the aorta and carotid sinus. Neurohormones (adrenaline and noradrenaline) bind to alpha-1 post-synaptic receptors on smooth muscle cells of the terminal arterioles, opening calcium channels and allowing Ca^{2+} ions

to enter cells. Post-synaptic alpha-2 and beta receptors also play a role, and several other hormonal systems exert an influence on microvessels [30], such as :
- angiotensin II (renin-angiotensin II-aldosterone system) which has a vasoconstrictor and stabilizing action;
- vasopressin (antidiuretic hormone) which responds to signals from the baroreceptors;
- the vasodilator action of kinin from the kallicrein-kinin-bradykinin system.

Endothelial cells regulate vessel diameter (bore size) and so influence both blood flow and pressure in a complex battery of mechanisms. A principle action is mediated by secretion of endothelium-derived relaxing factor (EDRF) discovered by Fruchgott, and identified as nitrogen dioxide [60]. The endothelium in turn interacts with neurohormones in a complex manner [78]. The following actions have been identified : inactivation of bradykinin, conversion of angiotensin I to II by converting enzyme, secretion of the vasoconstrictor endothelin and the vasodilator prostacyclin. All these actions impinge on parietal smooth muscle cells. The endothelium can thus be seen as an important effector organ for the regulation of blood flow in the microcirculation. It also modulates the shearing forces between blood and vessel walls (stress regulation).

Local factors

Locally acting mechanisms have particular importance at the terminal arterioles which are devoid of innervation, and so are less sensitive to the influences described above. There are considerable differences, though, from one organ to another. A reduction in oxygen partial pressure (PO_2) leads to a relaxation of smooth muscle cells, and hence vasodilatation. The main mediator here is adenosine. However, cerebral blood flow is not affected by this mechanism, but reacts rather to P_{CO_2} and H^+ ion concentration.

The myogenic reflex is triggered by stretching of smooth muscle cells (stretch activation) leading to vasoconstriction, especially in response to hyperpressure on the venous side of the microcirculatory unit. Various mediators have been identified including : a cellular sensor, endothelin and PO_2.

Another property of the microcirculation has been described recently by Intaglietta [37], which he refers to as vasomotion. It consists of cycles of vasoconstriction and vasodilation mainly occurring in arterioles originating in the forks of the microvessels (pace-maker effect). This activity is increased in certain metabolic and hemodynamic stress states. Loss of this property appears to be detrimental to tissue perfusion.

Finally, the contractions of lymphatic saccules also play a part in the local control of blood flow in the microcirculation.

Regulation of tissue exchange

The overall perfusion in the microcirculation unit depends on the resultant of the residual motor pressure and the extent of vasoconstriction of the terminal arterioles and precapillary arterioles (precapillary sphincters). The terminal arterioles are responsive to general influences, whereas the capillaries are more sensitive to local factors. Blood flow in the microcirculatory network can thus vary considerably from one territory to another, and in some areas permanent or temporary shut-down of the microcirculation can occur. This is frequently observed in muscles and skin where such processes represent an essential mechanism of regulation of volume and pressure in the arterial system. The venous side has more effect on blood volume via the blood storage properties of the venules. The arteriolar side via its vasomotor properties has more effect on pressure.

Exchange of gases, fluid and molecules between the blood and tissues is an essential property of the microcirculation unit. The alteration in hemodynamics in these tiny vessels (see below) leads to the formation of a slow moving circumferential layer of plasma, which favors exchange of substances between blood and tissues. This plasma layer is observed in nearly all vessels, but has particular importance in two vessel types:

- in the true capillaries where exchanges with tissues occur first with the plasma layer, and then as the bore narrows, with plasma and cells in contact with vessel walls (50 % of capillaries have a diameter below (5 µ). Exchange of gases takes place principally on the contact of red cells with vessel walls. These cells move in single file or in *rouleaux* in these narrow vessels. The capillary system is particularly sensitive to the perfusion pressure, and thus to arteriolar vasomotricity;

- venules where the sluggish flow favors exchanges between the plasma layer and tissues. Venous hyperpressure will clearly have an influence on this process.

Exchanges are therefore regulated essentially by pressure with an equilibrium between hydrostatic and oncotic pressures at the vessel wall *(Figure 2)*. Proper functioning of the lymphatic system is also required, with collection of fluid from atria and vesicles with their 3-6 per minute cyclic contractions.

Regulation of cellular exchange (microrheology)

Alteration in local hemodynamics

The Fahraeus effect is a characteristic property of the microcirculation, wich is manifest in vessels with diameters below 100 µ. Initially is characterized by a fall in hematocrit, which is much lower in microvessels. Blood flow

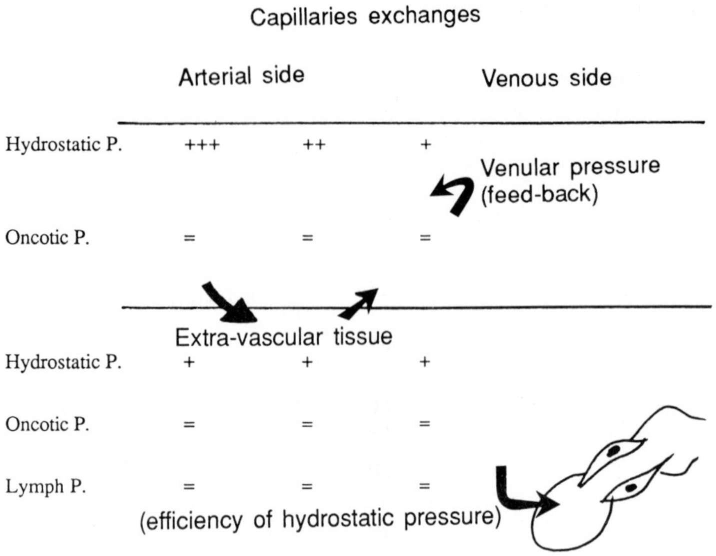

Capillaries exchanges

	Arterial side		Venous side
Hydrostatic P.	+++	++	+
			Venular pressure (feed-back)
Oncotic P.	=	=	=

Extra-vascular tissue

Hydrostatic P.	+	+	+
Oncotic P.	=	=	=
Lymph P.	=	=	=

(efficiency of hydrostatic pressure)

Figure 2. Tissue exchange : role of different pressures. Importance of a low pressure in the venulae.

is characterized by a central arrangement of red cells in discontinuous *rouleaux* separated by white cells and surrounded by a circumferential plasma layer which contains a significant proportion of platelets. Except in the true capillaries, this layer moves more slowly than the inner red cell stream which favors the restoration of a normal hematocrit at the output of the microcirculation [26]. The fall in hematocrit reduces viscosity, although this is sometimes increased by sedimentation and accumulation [25].

Leucocytes tend to move to the circumference in the plasma layer under chemotactic influences. In fact, the microcirculation appears to be the major site of action of leucocytes since blood flow is relatively slow, and is even further slowed as it meanders through the network [45]. The formation of *rouleaux* and aggregates of red cells further enhances the centrifugal movement of leucocytes [25].

There are, however, considerable regional differences in blood flow in the microcirculation in both normal and pathological circumstances. There is often and uneven distribution of cells at the vessel forks, and plasma tends to pass into the branch with the lower flow (plasma skimming effect) [65].

In the presence of hyperfibrinogenemia, for example, the increased aggregation of red cells with further hamper flow at vessel forks. In addition, it will favor stasis, especially in the post-capillary venules increasing the centrifugal movement of white cells and accelerating the passage of fluid across the vessel walls into tissues [26].

Behavior of blood cells

In order to pass through true capillaries, red cells must change their shape. Cell deformability depends on three factors: overall shape, membrane viscoelasticity and viscosity of cell contents. These parameters may be altered in various pathologies, the most notable being sickle cell anemia and diabetes. Leucocytes are 100 times more rigid than red cells [73], and can thus clog vessels with diameters under 20 μ. Normally, unlike red cells, they pass through arteriovenous anastomoses at a relatively high rate, which means that the microcirculation contains lower levels of white cells than does the general circulation [26]. However, a completely different situation arises under inflammatory conditions, when white cells move to the circumference of vessels tending to roll slowly along vessel walls. White cells normally only pass into tissues from the postcapillary venules. This is where flow is most sluggish and shear rates are lowest. Hematocrit is on the increase and may rise above normal due to sedimentation and accumulation. The mean velocity of leucocytes is at its lowest ebb in these vessels, and polymorphonuclear neutrophils (PMN), monocytes and lymphocytes readily move to the circumference and migrate across vessel walls thereby entering tissues.

These findings have important clinical implications. Under pathological conditions giving rise to venous hyperpressure or inflammation, white cells adhere and become activated on contact with vessel walls in the postcapillary venules and venules. White cells are sensitive to shear, and will only adhere if the shear-stress with the vessel walls is under 5 dynes/cm^2 [40], which is encountered in vessels where flow rates are low.

Endothelial cells and cellular adhesion

The endothelium has a normal hemostatic action mediated by an assortment of substances such as the platelet anti-aggregant, prostacyclin (PGI2), thrombomodulin which neutralizes thrombin, plasminogen activator (t-PA), and heparan sulfate which binds to antithrombin III. On the other hand, the endothelium can exhibit prothrombotic activity abetted by the presence of cytokines (IL1, IL6, TNF) and pathological factors such as oxygen-derived free radicals. The following processes have been described:
- alteration in the shape of endothelial cells, with the protruding cells forming gaps between cells [26];
- expression of integrins [15], ligands for leucocytes such as ICAM (lymphocytes), ILAM-1 (Polymorphonuclear and monocytes) and GMP-140 released from granules and expressed on the cell surface [28];
- secretion of a tissue factor, triggering the extrinsic coagulation pathway (factor VII pathway); secretion of von Willebrand factor, a red cell ligand [75,76]; PAI-1; platelet activating factor (PAF) [67]; interleukin 1 (IL1);

- reduction in anti-thrombotic activities.

In response to these changes, leucocytes adhere to and interact with the endothelium. The nature of these interactions which has only recently been uncovered appear to have considerable pathophysiological significance [34, 42].

Leucocyte activation is stimulated by :
- the presence of cytokine : Interleukin1, Interleukin6, tumor necrosis factor (TNF) [61];
- chemoattractants FLMP [51], C5a;
- agonists ADP [3], endotoxins, LTB4 with a direct action on PMN [51, 59], PAF [16, 67, 79];
- thrombin [80].

Activation is characterized biochemically by the expression of leu-CAM beta-integrins (CD11/CD18) [2, 61].

Interactions with endothelium are favored by stasis, and so tend to occur mainly in the post-capillary venules. The regulation of these processes is poorly understood, but 13-HODE and 23-HETES [7] are throught to have a stabilizing action, one with an activating and the other a deactivating effect. In addition, leucocytes appear to secrete their own adhesion inhibitor, LAI [84].

Activated monocytes in contact with the endothelium have enhanced procoagulant properties, secreting a tissue factor and expressing binding sites for fibrinogen and factors Xa and VIIa [1, 74] and PGE2 [72].

Red cells may also adhere to activated endothelium with von Willebrand factor as possible ligand [75].

Amplification in pathology

A whole repertoire of cell-mediated processes underlie the interactions between white cells and endothelium. For example, endothelial cells secrete PAF [13], and IL1. PMN produce PAF [69] and cathepsin G which also acts on platelets. The combination of cathepsin G and granulocyte elastase degrades heparin cofactor II, which then exhibits strong chemoattractant properties [36]. Amplification of LTB4 production by PMN is triggered by erythrocyte LTA4 [46, 71]. Platelets produce PAF and ADP which acts on PMN and other platelets. Monocytes produce PAF, IL1 and NAF [14]. Lastly, lymphocyte LIF influences adhesion of PMN [64].

It can be seen, therefore, that there is a strong link between ischemia and thrombosis. In ischemia, PMN activate endothelial cells via production of free radicals [41], and can bind factor Xa and fibrinogen to CR3 receptors [86]. They also have a vasoconstrictor action of the endothelium. Endothelial cells can bind factor Xa and produce fibrin, a property shared by monocytes. Various pathological conditions, of which diabetes is a prime example, stimulate these processes [66].

Such mechanisms play a crucial role in ischemia (PMN/endothelial interactions) and thrombosis (monocytes/endothelium/factor VII interactions) [55], and better understanding of these process will undoubtedly spur the development of new therapeutic strategies.

Investigations

Investigation of the microcirculation

In clinical practice, investigations are aimed at exploration of the structure and function of microvessels. In vasospastic disorders (Raynaud's syndrome, scleroderma), diabetes, and hypertension, the structure of the microvessels can be studied by periungual or conjunctival capillaroscopy along with the fluorescein permeability tests. This can be combined with digital plethysmography where the arterial pressure in the digits is measured before and after venous counterpressure.

In chronic arteriopathy of lower limbs, residual function of microvessels, especially after ischemia, can be explored by Doppler-Laser photometry which determines the flow rate of blood cells in a 1 mm^3 volume under the skin. Transcutaneous measurement of PO_2 is also employed. Determination of subcutaneous transit of labelled substances can be used to evaluate impairment of permeability and the origin of edema.

Investigation of microrheology

Direct investigation of blood cells has mostly been carried out in animals, and is not yet really feasible in man. Three main types of investigation have been employed.

Analysis of rheological factors in zones of stasis

Measurement of viscosity at low shear rates, which assesses the effects of aggregation of red cells, can give an *in vitro* estimate of potential rates of blood flow in post-capillary venules as well as in zones of stasis such as the vessels immediately after a stenosis or in ischemic regions. Such investigations are of value prior to surgical treatment of arteriopathy of the lower limbs, and in disorders of the venous system.

Deformability of blood cells

The deformability of red cells and leucocytes can be evaluated *ex vivo,* and has been the subject of a considerable body of research. There are marked an consistent alterations in erythrocyte deformability in sickle cell anemia, xerocytosis and poorly controlled diabetes, although in vascular disease, they are not so well established. Furthermore, the effects of the alteration in deformability are not easy to assess *in vivo*. For example, in sickle cell anemia, the decrease in deformability appears to have less pathological significance than the adhesion of cells to activated vessel walls, although it is clear that the two phenomena are related.

Leucocytes remain rigid after activation [5], and the reduced deformability of these cells has been implicated in some manifestations of vascular disease [52, 53].

Methods for analyzing cellular deformability such as timing passage through filters of graded pore size are not always interpretable as aggregates of cells can plug filter pores. This has now given rise to the notion of cellular filterability rather than deformability. The value of ektacytometry has also been questioned due to the extraphysiological conditions under which it is used, and its extreme sensitivity to intracellular viscosity.

Leucocyte activation

Methods for the evaluation of PMN and monocyte activation are being developed, and when available should throw more light on the role of these cells in ischemia and thrombosis. In the absence of acute inflammatory processes, plasma levels of elastase and myeloperoxidase are related to activation of PMN. The determination of the expression of leu-CAM beta-integrins on membranes can give an estimate of the proportion of activated circulating leucocytes (MAC 1, CR 3) [15]. Polymerization of actin [5, 23, 58], also reflects the state of activation or priming of leucocytes.

Another approach is to assess activation of coagulation at the surface of monocytes, by determination of factor Xa, the presence of derivatives of fibrin, and fibrinogen receptors [38, 43, 56].

The estimation of ischemia and thrombotic risk will undoubtedly benefit from further developments in these areas. From a pharmacological point of view, drugs acting on the endothelium and leucocytes and the interactions between them could then be devised [23].

Pathophysiology

Diseases of the microcirculation have a variety of causes, involving damage to the structure of, and impairments in vasomotricity of the microvessels. Rheological factors are involved to differing extents in such disorders, and much remains to be found out about their pathophysiological significance. However, they appear to be implicated in four main types of pathology.

Vasospastic disorders

Raynaud's syndrome is essentially a disorder of vasomotricity, and rheological parameters are usually normal in this condition. However, in acrocyanosis, acrosyndromes secondary to risk factors and in scleroderma, microrheological factors play a role in the inflammatory syndrome.

High blood pressure

Essential hypertension can be viewed as a model of abnormal pressure and flow regulation in terminal arterioles. The advent of calcium blockers in the treatment of high blood pressure has highlighted the role of peripheral resistance under this condition. High blood pressure is accompanied by an increase in plasma viscosity due to the raised fibrinogen levels and the hyperaggregation of red cells. These disorders illustrate the significance of the microcirculation unit, not only for its resistive properties, but also for the balance between rheological and plasma factors within microvessels.

Rheological diseases

Red cell diseases

Sickle cell anemia is characterized by a disorder in deformability of red cells, also observed in the heterozygotes. It is due to cellular dehydration, and an increased intra-cellular hemoglobin concentration, enhanced by attachment of hemoglobin S granules to the plasma membrane. In fact, this defect in deformability appears less deleterious than the increased tendency of these altered red cells to adhere to the damaged or activated endothelium giving rise to microvascular thromboses.
Hereditary familial xerocytosis is characterized by a dehydration of red cells due to a massive influx of Ca^{2+} ions. This rheological disorder resulting from an increase in intracellular viscosity is readily visualized by ektacytometry.

Hyperviscosity syndromes

Various syndromes of plasma or erythrocyte hyperviscosity secondary to hematological diseases such as Vaquez polyglobulia and dysproteinemias have been described. In shock, there is a massive adhesion of leucocytes to the endothelium especially in the adult respiratory distress syndrome (ARDS) [63]. Mention should also be made of the primary hyperviscosity syndromes, largely idiopathic, which are revealed by an impairment of the microcirculation especially in the inner ear with repercussions on hearing. In this case, there is a chronic contraction of plasma volume, sometimes accompanied by elevations in hematocrit and fibrinogen. The mechanism is poorly understood, although it impairs the microcirculation. It may have some relation to hypertension since calcium blockers and drugs which reduce peripheral resistance improve the condition.

Vascular diseases and microcirculation

Disorders of the microcirculation are fundamental to vascular disease both from a pathophysiological and therapeutic standpoint.

Venous disease

Chronic superficial venous insufficiency induces a progressive impairment in the microcirculation on the venous side, leading to venous hyperpressure [8]. The venules are the sites of disorders of permeability, resulting in edema, contraction of plasma volume with concomitant hyperviscosity and enhanced aggregation of red cells. These initially local disorders tend to become disseminated throughout the circulation. Progressive inhibition of flow in post-capillary venules also favors adhesion of leucocytes and ulceration.

Arterial disease

Atherosclerosis, an inflammatory and deforming disease of arterial walls, is accompanied by generalized rheological disorders. Risk factors for atheroma such as high blood pressure and diabetes [38] tend to induce bouts of inflammation accompanied by increased secretion of cytokines. The rheological disturbances can be largely accounted for by the hyperfibrinogenemia, the contraction of plasma volume stemming from the enhanced vascular permeability and the activation of leucocytes and endothelial cells [20]. In addition, abnormalities in membrane lipids [23] decrease the deformability and enhance the priming of circulating cells. A variety of compensatory mechanisms tend to conceal the rheological disorders which only become apparent where there is a defect in driving pressure and flow in the large systemic vessels harboring atherosclerotic plaques. Three areas tend to be affected:

- zones of stenosis: platelets are activated around plaques essentially as a result of shear stress. In the stagnant post-stenosed zone, the low flow rates favor adhesion of leucocytes to the activated endothelium thereby triggering coagulation [19];

- post-stenosis ischemic zones : the initial studies of Bagge [4, 5], Engler [17] and Gaethgens [27] have demonstrated adhesion of leucocytes to the endothelium in ischemic vessels. This significant phenomenon blocks the microcirculation (no-reflow effect) [31, 35, 53] via local diffusion of cytokines and free radicals, and especially LTB4 [29]. Vasomotor disorders thus develop in parallel with the ischemia [32];

- peri-thrombotic zones : adherence of cells to vessel walls in peri-thrombotic regions also tends to aggravate the lesions.

Coronary disease and myocardial infarction also lead to rheological disorders [18]. One index of infarction is represented by the leucocyte count [24, 33, 87], but it can also be assessed from the adhesive properties of these cells [70], and their state of activation [47]. The rigidity of leucocytes indicated by filtration tests is related to their degree of activation [12, 54]. In animal studies, depletion or inactivation of leucocytes using monoclonal antibodies has been shown to reduce the area of ischemia [57, 62, 68].

Activation and rheological changes in leucocytes are also observed in stroke [11, 21, 22, 81, 83].

Thus it can be seen that although the microrheological alterations may not be the cause of the vascular obstruction from atheroma or platelet aggregation, they do tend to make the situation worse [10]. Besides platelet behavior and vasomotor factors, rheological factors do, therefore, need to be taken into account in such conditions.

Thrombosis

Microrheological factors play a dual role in thrombotic processes. A thrombus can form on damaged and activated endothelium in zones where blood flow is low. The coagulant properties of blood cells, especially those of monocytes may be translocated, inducing venous thromboses [19, 55, 56] or disseminated intravascular coagulation [43].

Conclusion

The microcirculation is regulated in a complex manner by a combination of vasomotor and flow control mechanisms. The characteristics of the microcirculation vary from territory to territory and from organ to organ, but its role in a number of pahtological processes is now beginning to be unravelled.

Microrheology is intimately bound up with the microcirculation in both health and disease, and is receiving increasing attention in view of its relationship with inflammatory processes and microcirculatory hemodynamics. The characteristics of blood flow in the microvessels thus represents a potential target for new therapeutic agents, especially those designed for the treatment and prevention of vascular disease.

References

1. Altieri DC, Bader R, Mannuci PM *et al*. Oligospecificity of the cellular adhesion receptor MAC-1 encompasses an inducible recognition specificity for fibrinogen. J Cell Biol, 1988; 107 : 1893-1900.
2. Arnaout MA. Structure and function of the leukocyte adhesion molecules CD11/CD18. Blood, 1990; 75 : 1037-1050.
3. Axtell RA, Sandborg RR, Smolen JE *et al*. Exposure of human neutrophils to exogenous nucleotides causes elevation in intracellular calcium, transmembrane calcium fluxes and an alteration of a cytosolic factor resulting in enhanced superoxyde production in response to FLMP and arachidonic acid Blood, 1990; 75 : 1324-1332.
4. Bagge U, Amundson B, Lauritzen C. White blood cells deformability and plugging of skeletal muscle capillaries in haemorrhagic shock. Acta Physiol Scand, 1980; 108 : 159-163.
5. Bagge U. Granulocyte rheology. Blood Cells, 1976; 2 : 481-490.
6. Belloc F, Vincendeau P, Freyburger G *et al*. A flow cytometry study of the activation of polymorphonuclear cells. J Leuk Biol, (in press).
7. Buchanan MR, Bastida E. Endothelium and underlying membrane reactivity with platelets, leukocytes and tumor cells : regulation by the lipoxygenase-derived fatty acid metabolites, 13-HODE and HETES. Med Hypotheses, 1988; 27 : 317-325.
8. Chabanel A, Glacet-Bernard A, Lelong F, *et al*. Increased blood cell aggregation in retinal vein occlusion. Br J Haemat, 1990; 75 : 127-131.
9. Casillas JM, Didier JP, Lucet A *et al*. Adaptation cardio-respiratoire, métabolique et microcirculatoire au cours de l'artériopathie oblitérante des membres inférieurs. Sem Hôp Paris, 1990; 66 : 333-337.
10. Ciufetti G, Mercuri M, Rizzo MT *et al*. Human leukocyte rheology and tissue ischaemia. Eur J Clin Invest, 1989; 19 : 323-327.
11. Ciuffetti G, Mercuri M, Mannarino E *et al*. Leucocyte rheology in the early stages of ischaemic stroke. Klin Wochenschr, 1989; 67 : 762-763.
12. Ciufetti G, Bellomo G, Mercuri M *et al*. Leucocyte rheology in controlled coronary ischaemia. Int J Cardiol, 1989; 193-198.
13. Coëffier E, Delautier D, Le Couedic JP *et al*. Cooperation between platelets and neutrophils for PAF-acether (Platelet-activating Factor) formation. J Leuk Biol, 1990; 47 : 23-243.

14. Colditz I, Zwahlen R, Dewald B, Baggiolini M. *In vivo* inflammatory activity of neutrophil-activating factor, novel chemotactic peptide derived from human monocytes. Amer. J. Pathol., 1989; 134 : 755-760.
15. Detmers PA, Wright SD. Adhesion-promoting receptors of leukocytes. Current Op. Immunol., 1988; 1 : 10-15.
16. Dillon PK, Fitzpatrick MF, Ritter AB *et al*. Effect of platelet-activating factor on leukocyte adhesion to microvascular endothelium. Inflammation, 1988; 12 : 563-570.
17. Engler RL, Schmidt-Schönbein GW, Pavelee RS. Leukocyte capillary plugging in myocardial ischaemia and reperfusion in the dog. Am J Pathol, 1983; 111 : 98-111.
18. Engler RL, Dahlgreen MD, Peterson MA *et al*. Accumulation of polymorphonuclear leukocytes during experimental myocardial ischemia. Heart Circ Physiol, 1986; 20 : H93-H100.
19. Ernst E, Hammerschmidt DE, Bagge U *et al*. Leukocytes and the risk of ischaemic diseases. JAMA, 1987; 257 : 2318-2324.
20. Enrst E, Matrai A. Altered red and white blood cell rheology in type II diabetes. Diabetes, 1986; 35 : 1412-1415.
21. Ernst E, Matrai A, Paulsen F. Leukocyte rheology in recent stroke. Stroke, 1987; 18 : 59-62.
22. Ernst E, Matrai A, Marshall M. Blood rheology in patients with transient ischemic attacks. Stroke, 1988; 19 : 634-636.
23. Freyburgher G, Gin H, Heape A *et al*. Phospholipid and fatty acid composition of erythrocytes in type I and type II diabetes. Metabolism, 1989; 38 : 673-678.
24. Friedman GD, Klatsky AL, Siegelaub AB. The leukocyte count at a predictor of myocardial infarction. N Engl J Med, 1974; 290 : 1275-1278.
25. Gaethghens P. Microvascular flow disturbances : rheological aspects. In Manabe H *et al.*, Microcirculation in circulatory disorders. Springer Verlag, 1988.
26. Gaethgens P. Pathways and interactions of white cells in the microcirculation. In K Messmert *et al.*, Progress in applied microcirculation. Karger, 1987.
27. Gaethgens SP, Ley K, Pries AR *et al*. Actual interaction between leukocytes and microvascular blood flow. Prog Appl Microcirc, 1985; 7 : 15-28.
28. Geng JG, Bevilacqua MP, Moore KL *et al*. Rapid neutrophil adhesion to activated endothelium mediated by GMP-140. Nature, 1990; 343 : 757-758.
29. Goldman G, Welbourn R, Paterson IS *et al*. Ischemia-induced neutrophil activation and diapedesis is lipoxygenase dependent. Surgery, 1990; 107 : 428-433.
30. Granger HJ, Schelling ME, Lewis RE *et al*. Physiology and pathobiology of the microcirculation. Am J Otolaryngol, 1988; 9 : 264-277.
31. Granger DN, Benoit JN, Suzuki M *et al*. Leukocyte adherence to venular endothelium during ischemia-reperfusion. Am J Physiol, 1989; 257 : G683-G688.
32. Grossman HJ, Zambetis M. Leucocyte-induced endothelium-dependent vasodilatation and post-ischaemic vasospasm in the isolated rat superior mesenteric artery. Br J Exp Path, 1989; 70 : 515-523.
33. Haines AP, Howarth D, North WRS *et al*. Haemostatic variables and the outcome of myocardial infarction. Thromb. Haemostas, 1983; 50 : 800-803.
34. Harlan JM. Leukocyte-endothelial interactions. Blood, 1985; 65 : 513-525.
35. Hernandez LA, Grisham MB, Twohig B *et al*. Role of neutrophils in ischemia-reperfusion-induced microvascular injury. Am J Physiol, 1987; 253 : H699-H703.

36. Hoffman M, Pratt CW, Brown RL et al. Heparin cofactor II-proteinase reaction products exhibit neutrophil chemoattractant activity. Blood, 1989; 73 : 1682-1685.
37. Intaglietta M. Vasomotion and flow modulation in the microcirculation. *In Progress in applied microcirculation* Vol 15. M Intaglietta Ed, 1 Vol, Karger 1989.
38. Jude B, Watel A, Fontaine O et al. Distinctive feature of procoagulant response of monocytes from diabetic patients. Haemostasis, 1989; 19 : 65-73.
39. Larcan A. *In Microcirculation et hémorhéologie*. A Larcan, JF Stoltz, Eds, 1 Vol, Masson 1970.
40. Lawrence MB, Smith CW, Eskin SG et al. Effect of venous shear stress on CD18-mediated neutrophil adhesion to cultured endothelium. Blood, 1990; 75 : 227-237.
41. Lewis MS, Whatley RE, Cain P et al. Hydrogen peroxide stimulates the synthesis of platelet activating factor by endothelium and induces endothelial cell-dependent neutrophil adhesion. J. Clin Invest, 1988; 82 : 2045-2055.
42. Lipowsky HH, House SD, Firrell JC. Leukocyte endothelium adhesion and microvascular hemodynamics. Adv Exp Med Biol, 1988; 242 : 85-93.
43. Luscher E. Activated leukocytes and the haemostatic system. Rev. Inf. Diseases, 1987; 9 : 5546-5557.
44. Manabe BW. Microcirculation in circulatory disorders. Manabe H, Zweifach BW, Messmer K Eds, 1 Vol. Springer-Verlag, 1988.
45. Mayrowitz HN, Kang SJ, Herscovici B et al. Leukocyte adherence initiation in skeletal muscle capillaries and venules. Microvasc Res, 1987; 33 : 22-34.
46. McGee JE, Fitzpatrick FA. Erythrocyte-neutrophil interactions : formation of leukotriene B4 by transcellular biosynthesis. Proc Natl Acad Sci USA, 1986; 83 : 1349-1353.
47. Mehta J. Dinerman J, Mehta P et al. Neutrophil function in ischemic heart disease. Circulation, 1989; 79 : 549-556.
48. Messmer K, Hammersen F. Microcirculation and inflammation : vessel wall-inflammatory cells-mediator interaction. *In Progress in applied microcirculation*, vol 12. Messmer Ed, 1 Vol Karger, 1987.
49. Messmer K, Hammersen. Cerebral microcirculation. In Progress in applied microcirculation vol 16, Messmer K, Hammersen F Eds, 1 Vol Karger, 1990.
50. Mortillaro NA. The physiology and pharmacology of the microcirculation, Vol 1. N. Mortillaro A. Ed., 1 Vol. Academic Press, 1983.
51. Nagai K, Katori M. Possible changes in the leukocyte membrane as a mechanism of leukocyte adhesion to the venular walls induced by leukotrien B4 and FLMP in the microvasculature of the hamster cheek pouch. Int. Microcirc J Clin Exp, 1988; 7 : 305-314.
52. Nash GB, Jones JG, Mikita J et al. Methods and theory for analysis of flow of white cell subpopulations through micropore filters. Brit Haemat J, 1988; 70 : 165-170.
53. Nash GB, Thomas PRS, Dormandy JA. Abnormal flow properties of white blood cells in patients with severe ischaemia of the leg. Brit Med J, 1988; 296-302.
54. Nash GB, Christopher B, Morris AJR et al. Changes in the flow properties of white cells after acute myocardial infarction. Br Heart J, 1989; 62 : 329-334.
55. Nygaard OP, Unneberg K, Reikeras O, Osterud B. Thromboplastin activity of blood monocytes after hip replacement. Scand J Clin Lab Invest, 1990; 50 : 183-186.
56. Ollivier V, Sheibani A, Chollet-Martin S et al. Monocyte procoagulant activity and membrane-associated D-Dimer after knee replacement surgery. Thromb Res, 1989; 55 : 179-185.

57. O'Neill PG, Charlat ML, Michael LH et al. Influence of neutrophil depletion on myocardial function and flow after reversible ischemia. Am J. Physiol, 1989; 256 : H341-H351.
58. Packman CH, Lichtman MA. Activation of neutrophils : measurement of actin conformational changes by flow cytometry. Blood cells, 1990; 16.
59. Palmblad J, Lindström P, Lerner R. Leukotrien B4 induced hyperadhesiveness of endothelial cells for neutrophils. Bioch Bioph Res Comm, 1990; 166 : 848-851.
60. Palmer RMJ, Ferrige AG, Moncada S. Nitric oxide release accounts for the biological activity of endothelium-derived relaxing factor. Nature, 1987; 327 : 524-526.
61. Pober JS. Cytoline-mediated activation of vascular endothelium. Am J. Pathol, 1988; 133 : 426-433.
62. Romson JL, Hook BG, Steven BS et al. Reduction of the extent of ischemic myocardial injury by neutrophil depletion in the dog. Circulation, 1983; 67 : 1016-1023.
63. Rossignon MD, Khayat D, Royer C et al. Functional and metabolic activity of polymorphonuclear leukocytes from patients with adult respiratory distress syndrome : results of a randomized double-blind placebo-controlled study on the activity of prostaglandin E1. Anesthesiology, 1990; 72 : 276-281.
64. Schainberg H, Borish L, King M et al. Leukocyte inhibitory factor stimulates neutrophil-endothelial cell adhesion. J. Immunol. 1988; 141 : 3055-3060.
65. Secomb TW, Fleischman GF, Papenfuss HD et al. Effects of reduced perfusion and hematocrit on flow distribution in capillary networks. In Messmer K, ref. 48, pp 205-211.
66. Setiadi H, Wautier JL, Courillon-Mallet A et al. Increased adhesion to fibronectin and MO-1 expression by diabetic monocytes. J Immunol., 1987; 138 : 3230-3234.
67. Shalit M, Dabiri GA, Southwick FS. Platelet-activating factor both stimulates and «primes» human polymorphonuclear leukocyte actin filament assembly. Blood, 1987; 70 : 1921-1927.
68. Simpson PJ, Todd III RF, Fantone JC et al. Reducation of experimental canine myocardial reperfusion injury by a monoclonal antibody (anti-Mol, anti-CD11b) that inhibits leukocyte adhesion. J Clin Invest, 1988; 81 : 624-629.
69. Sisson JH, Prescott SM, McIntyre TM et al. Production of platelet-activating factor by stimulated human polymorphonuclear leukocytes. J Immunol, 1987; 138 : 3918-3926.
70. Smith BD, Thomas JL, Gillespie JA. Abnormal erythrocyte endothelial adherence in ischemic heart disease. Clin Hemorh, 1990; 10 : 241-253.
71. Stern A, Serhan CN. Human red cells enhance the formation of 5-lipoxygenase-derived products by neutrophils. Free Rad Res Comms, 1989; 7 : 335-339.
72. Takayama TK, Miller C, Szabo G. Elevated tumor necrosis factor production concomitant to elevated prostaglandin E2 production by trauma patients' monocytes. Arch Surg, 1990; 125 : 29-35.
73. Thompson TN, La celle PL, Cokelet GR. Perturbation of red blood cell flow in small tubes by white blood cells. Pflügers Arch, 1989; 413 : 372-377.
74. Trezzini C, Jungi TW, Kuhnert P et al. Fibrinogen association with human monocytes : evidence for constitutive expression of fibrinogen receptors and for involvement of MAC-1 (CD18, CR3) in the binding. Bioch Bioph Res Comms, 1988; 156 : 477-484.
75. Tsai HM, Sussman II, Nagel RL et al. Desmopressin induces adhesion of normal human erythrocytes to the endothelial surface of a perfused microvascular preparation. Blood, 1990; 75 : 261-265.

76. Tsai HM, Nagel RL, Hachter VB *et al*. Multimeric composition of endothelial cell-derived von Willebrand factor. Blood, 1989; 73 : 2074-2076.
77. Tsuchiya M. Microcirculation. An update, Vol 1. M Tsuchiya, Asano M, Mishima Y, Oda M. Eds. 1 Vol., Excerpta Medica 1987.
78. Vanhoutte PM. Endothelium and control of vascular function. Hypertension, 1989, 13, 658-667.
79. Vercellotti GM, Yin HQ, Gustafson KS *et al*. Platelet-activating factor primes neutrophil responses to agonists : role in promoting neutrophil-mediated endothelial damage. Blood, 1988; 71 : 1100-1107.
80. Vercellotti GM, Wickham NWR, Gustafson KS *et al*. Thrombin-treated endothelium primes neutrophil functions : inhibition by platelet-activating factor receptor antagonists. J Leuk Biol, 1989; 45 : 483-490.
81. Vermes I, Strik F. Altered leukocyte rheology in patients with chronic cerebrovascular disease. Stroke, 1988; 19 : 631-633.
82. Vicaut E. Paramètres fondamentaux dans la physiologie de la microcirculation. STV, 1990; 2 : 65-71.
83. Violi F, Rasura M, Alessandri C *et al*. Leukocyte response in patients suffering from acute stroke. Stroke, 1988; 19 : 1283-1284.
84. Wheeler ME, Luscinskas FW, Bevilacqua MP, Gimbrone Jr MA. Cultured human endothelial cells stimulated with cytokines or endotoxin produce an inhibitor of leukocyte adhesion. J Clin Invest, 1988; 82 : 1211-1218.
85. Wiedeman MP. An introduction to microcirculation, 1 vol. Wiedeman MP, Tuma RF, Mayrovitz HN, Eds Vol 1. Academic Press, 1981.
86. Wright SD, Weitz JJ, Huang AJ *et al*. Complement receptor type three (CD 11b/CD 18) of human polymorphonuclear leukocytes recognizes fibrinogen. Proc Natl Acad Sci USA, 1988; 85 : 7734-7738.
87. Zalokar JB, Richard JL, Claude JR. Leukocyte count, smoking and myocardial infarction. New Eng J Med, 1981; 304 : 465-468.

2

Ω-3 fatty acids and microcirculation

G. Bruckner

Department of Clinical Sciences, University of Kentucky, USA.

Abstract

Three studies were conducted to determine the effects of different fats on blood flow in peripheral blood vessels, the type of dietary fat which has the greatest effect on peripheral blood flow and the effect of supplemented dietary vitamin E on the microcirculation. In normolipidemic adults, dietary fats rich in Ω-3 vs. Ω-9 fatty acid significantly increased nailfold capillary blood cell velocities. Hyperlipidemic adults responded to fats rich in Ω-3 and Ω-6 fatty acids with increases in capillary blood cell velocities. These changes in hyperlipidemia were persistent after a one month washout period. Geriatric normolipidemic individuals only showed significant increased blood flow velocities following Ω-3 fatty acid and vitamin E supplementation. This data suggests that Ω-3 and Ω-6 fatty acids, with adequate antioxidants, most likely increase peripheral capillary blood flow by altering vascular tone and blood viscosity. Furthermore, Ω-3 fatty acids without adequate antioxidant present may be detrimental with regard to peripheral capillary flow.

Introduction

Cardiovascular disease is one of the most significant dietary related health problems in the United States of America [1]. During the past decade a great deal of progress has been made toward defining the role of dietary fats and hypercholesterolemia in the pathogenesis of arteriosclerosis [2] and this, along with more public nutrition education, may be related to the observed steady decline in morbidity and mortality from cardiovascular disease [3]. The etiology of cardiovascular disease is multifaceted and although many findings support the involvement of dietary fat and cholesterol in atherogenesis [1, 4], the mechanisms involved are not clearly understood. For example, it is known that different fatty acid isomers, Ω-3 vs. Ω-6 20 carbon fatty acids, can elicit completely different vascular responses as evidenced by the Greenland Eskimo studies and subsequent reports by Dyerberg and Bang [5] and others [6-9]. Recent work by Grundy [10] also suggests that various monounsaturated fatty acids can have different cholesterol-lowering effects. Therefore, it is evident that a number of factors in addition to serum cholesterol are involved in the etiology of cardiovascular disease, e.g. blood flow, platelet endothelial interaction, lipid hydroperoxides, etc. Changes in capillary blood flow have been noted in subjects with atherosclerotic disease [11], however it is not clear whether these changes contribute to the etiology of the disease or are the consequence of the disease process. Changes in blood flow and platelet-endothelial cell interactions have been implicated to directly influence atherogenesis [12]. We postulate that the interactions of circulating lipids with endothelial surfaces depend in part on the rate of blood flow. The constant exposure of the endothelium to various blood components, including prooxidants such as fatty acid peroxides or oxidized derivatives of cholesterol, may damage or alter a number of endothelial cell functions, e.g. synthesis of antiaggregatory vasodilators (prostacyclin), endothelial cell permeability and/or platelet endothelial cell adhesion. It is possible that these lipids, particularly the oxidized forms, along with the products of cellular metabolism, may elicit greater cellular damage in slower flowing vessels. This may be due to prolonged contact with these surfaces, resulting in an increased chance for initiation of lesion development. Therefore, it is important to better understand the effects of different fatty acids on blood flow. Moreover, due to the differing susceptibility of various fatty acids to oxidative reactions it is important to determine the degree to which these fatty acids are oxidized and their effects on events associated with microcirculatory changes and atherogenesis. Our ongoing studies are designed to help us better understand 1) the effects of different fats on blood flow in peripheral blood vessels and the underlying mechanism involved, 2) the amount and type of dietary fatty acid which has the greatest effect on peripheral blood flow, and 3) the effect of the dietary antioxidant vitamin E on the microcirculation.

Methods and results

Three studies have been conducted to assess the effects of Ω-3 fatty acid supplementation on microcirculatory changes.

Study number 1

Twelve normolipidemic male subjects (cholesterol <220, triglycerides <250) were recruited for the study aged 18-40. The study was a parallel design with no crossover. Subjects were randomly allocated to fish oil (Ω-3 fatty acid*) or olive oil supplemented groups at 1.5 g oil/10, kg Bwt/day. All capsules contained 1 I.U. vitamin E/g oil. Nailfold capillary blood cell velocities were measured before and after 3 weeks of supplementation as well as biochemical lipid parameters (cholesterol, triglycerides, and high density lipoproteins). These results and the microcirculatory methodologies have been previously published [7] and are depicted in *Figure 1*. Capillary blood cell velocity was significantly increased by fish vs. olive oil supplementation. No washout measurements were made.

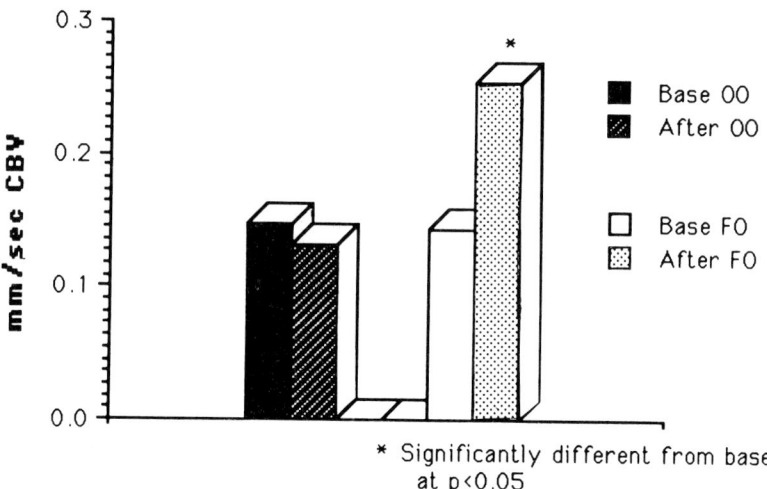

* Significantly different from base at p<0.05

Figure 1. Changes in nailfold capillary blood cell velocities before and after three weeks supplementation with olive or fish oil at 1.5 g oil/kg Bwt/day.

Study number 2.

Thirty-two hyperlipidemic (cholesterol 220 mg/dl and triglycerides 250 mg/dl) male subjects aged 18-55 were recruited and randomly allocated

---

(*) Maxepa®.

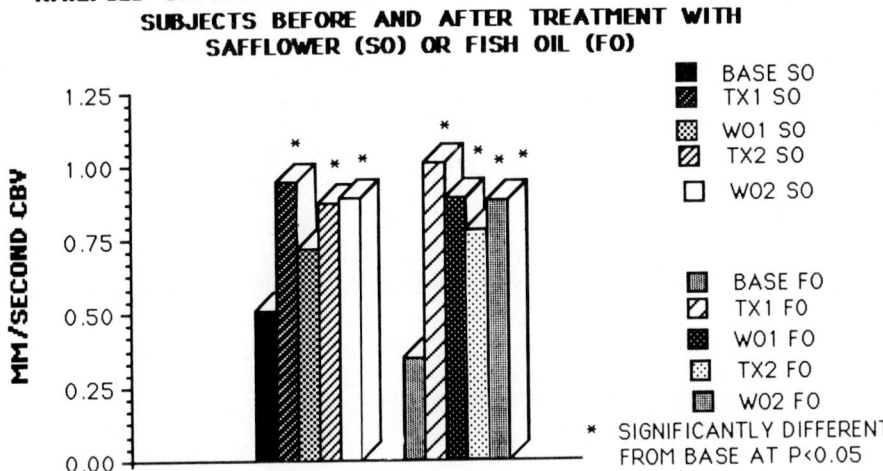

Figure 2. Changes in nailfold capillary blood cell velocities before (base), after two months supplementation with fish or safflower oil (TX$_1$), following one month washout prior to next treatment regimen (WO$_1$), and after treatment two (TX$_2$) or washout 2 (WO$_2$).

to four treatment groups; fish oil and oat bran, fish oil (Ω-3 fatty acid) and wheat bran, safflower oil and oat branch or safflower oil and wheat bran. Oils were supplemented at 1.5 g oil/10 kg Bwt/day and bran at approximately 10 g total fiber/subject/day. The experimental design was a crossover design balanced for residual effects. Each subject therefore received each treatment combination over the course of one year. Baseline or washout measurements for capillary blood cell velocity were determined on all subjects prior to and after two months of treatment. All subjects discontinued supplements for one month washout before starting the next regimen. As shown in *Figure 2*, capillary blood cell velocity was increased significantly by fish oil and safflower oil supplementation over baseline. Fiber did not contribute to capillary blood cell velocity changes. Capillary blood cell velocity never returned to the original baseline values after either fish or safflower oil intervention, although serum fatty acids returned to normal values after a one month washout period (data not shown).

Study number 3

Forty normolipidemic (cholesterol <220, triglycerides <250) male geriatric subjects (55-70) were recruited through the Sanders-Brown Aging Center at the University of Kentucky. They were randomly allocated to 4 groups as follows: Purified fish oil product containing approximately 50 % Ω-3 fatty

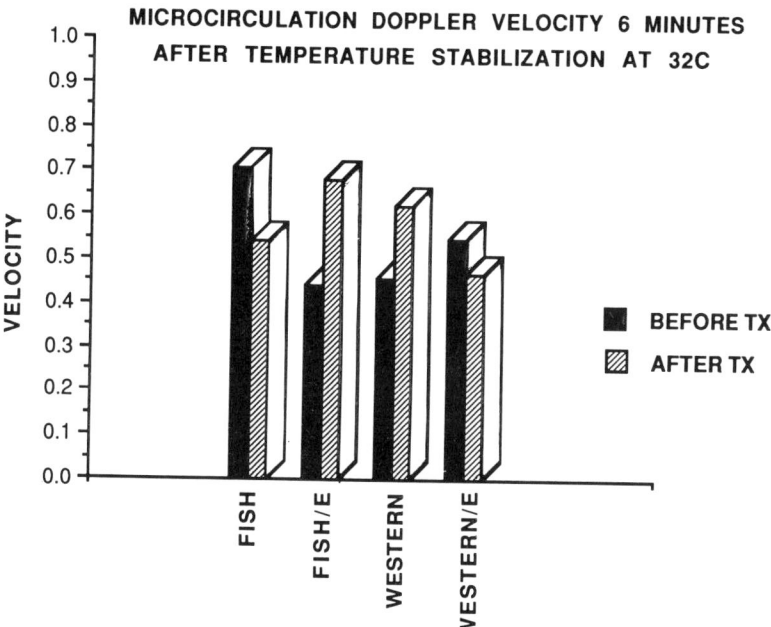

Figure 3. Changes in subdermal blood flow velocity as measured by laser doppler in Hz units before and after 4 weeks supplementation with the various oils with or without 800 I.U. Vit E/day. All oils supplemented at 1.5 g/10 kg Bwt/day. Only fish/E after TX is significantly different from before TX at p .05.

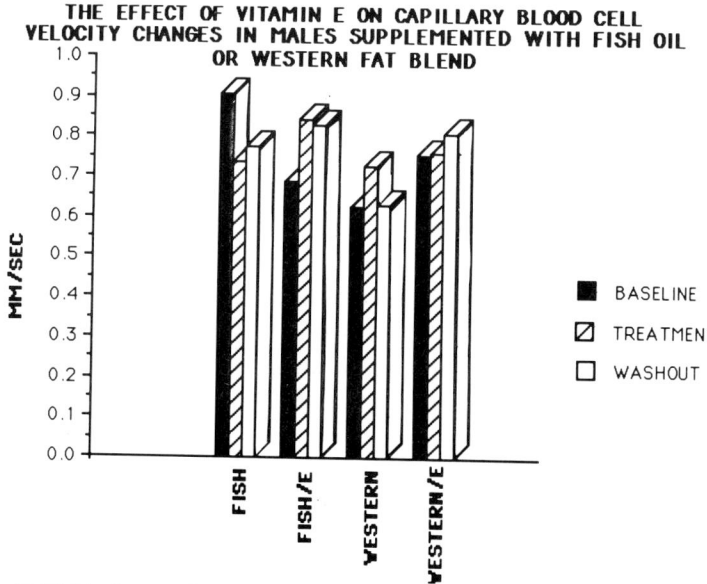

Figure 4. Nailfold changes in geriatric male subjects supplemented with various oils for 4 weeks (treatment) at 1.5 g/10 kg Bwt/day with or without 800 I.U./day vitamin E. Washout measurements were conducted 4 months after supplements were discontinued.

acid with or without vitamin E, and Western diet fat blend with or without vitamin E (a mixture of lard, tallow and corn oil to mimic average daily fat intake in US population). All oils were given at 1.5 g/10 kg Bwt/day. Vitamin E supplemented at 800 I.U./day. Laser doppler flow and capillary blood cell velocity measurements were made before and after two months of supplementation and followings two months washout. The fish oil with vitamin E increased velocity of subdermal and CBV as measured by laser doppler and videomicroscopy (see *Figures 3 and 4)*. However, the fish treatment alone decreased CBV from that noted for baseline and the other treatments which did not result in notable changes.

Blood pressure, serum lipids and blood viscosity were measured as previously reported [7] in all three studies.

Discussion

Ω-3 fatty acid related factors which may affect peripheral microcirculation are blood pressure, blood viscosity and vascular tone *(Figure 5)*. Systemic

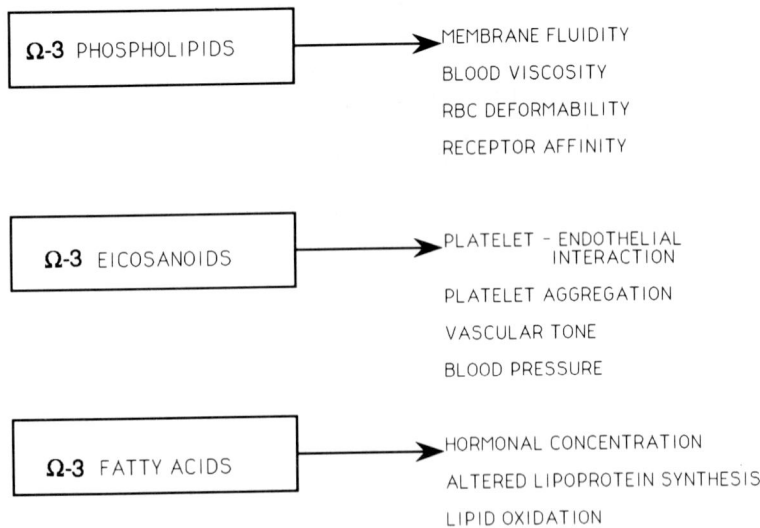

Figure 5. Ω-3 fatty acid may alter vascular responses via incorporation into phospholipids and/or subsequent release as eicosanoid precursors or perhaps directly by alteration of hormonal, lipoprotein or lipid peroxide synthesis.

Ω-3 fatty acids and microcirculation

blood pressure was measured in all these studies with no significant changes noted prior to or after oil supplementation. Additionally one would expect increased capillary blood cell velocity to be associated with increased blood pressure changes however, other investigators have demonstrated a decrease in systemic pressure following fish oil intervention [13].

Blood viscosity was measured in these studies using a capillary viscometer. There were no significant changes noted for plasma or whole blood using this method to determine blood viscosity, however, these measurements may differ from the results of others using a cone viscometer [14]. Both methods should be employed in future studies to help define these differences.

Our studies suggest that in humans, increased capillary blood cell velocity is most likely due to changes in precapillary vascular tone, i.e. vasodilatation, however, it is not clear what events bring about these changes *(Figure 6)*.

Changes in vascular tone may be altered by eicosanoid ratios (TXA_3/PGI_3; TXA_2/PGI_2) [15, 16], hormone concentrations, membrane structural changes and/or receptor agonist binding.

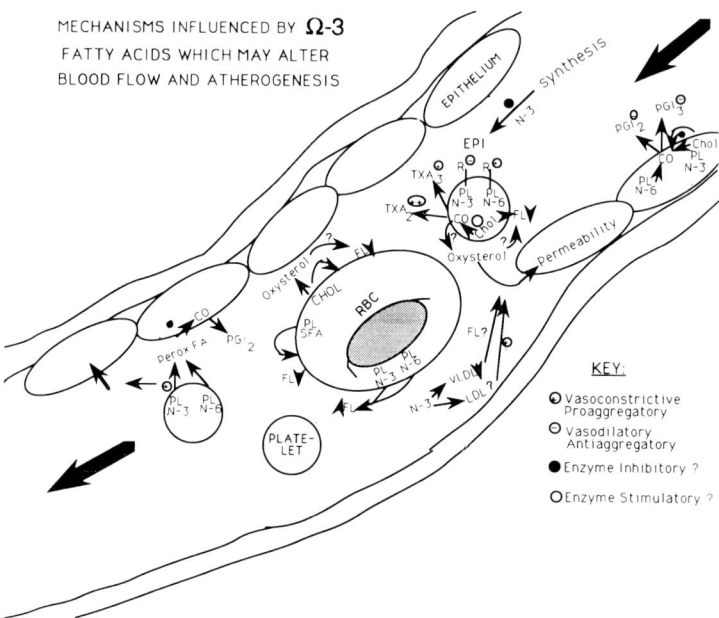

Figure 6. Ω-3 fatty acid may alter blood flow and atherogenesis by mechanism favoring the promotion of antiaggregatory and vasodilatory eicosanoids or altering membrane fluidity. These events may be altered by membrane viscosity and changes in circulating lipids and lipoproteins.

As depicted in *Figure 6,* we hypothesize that events which alter lipid peroxidation, eicosanoid production or membrane fluidity may alter vascular hemodynamics through a number of mechanisms. For example, if cholesterol is incorporated into platelet membranes, the increased production of vasoconstrictive eicosanoids (TXA_2) might be stimulated. Furthermore, cholesterol may decrease fluidity of the platelet and RBC membrane. We also speculate that cholesterol oxides may be produced from oxygenase activities which could lead to further vascular damage due to increased endothelial cell permeability. Ω-3 fatty acids may alter these events by favoring the production of vasodilatory eicosanoids and decreasing membrane fluidity, provided that these highly oxidizable lipids are protected by adequate antioxidants.

It is also possible that subtle insignificant individual changes in each of the three variables i.e. blood pressure, blood viscosity and vascular tone when combined may contribute to the significant changes which we have noted as increased capillary blood cell velocity after intervention with dietary Ω-3 or Ω-6 fatty acids. Additionally as suggested by the results of study number 3, the antioxidant status of the individual may determine if the addition of dietary unsaturated fatty acids is beneficial or detrimental to changes in peripheral microcirculation.

References

1. Surgeon General's Report on Nutrition and Health, US Department of Health and Human Services, 1988; DHHS No. 88-5021.
2. St Clair RW. Pathogenesis of the Atherosclerotic Lesion : Current Concepts of Cellular and Biochemical Events. Recent Advances in Arterial Diseases : Atherosclerosis, Hypertension, and Vasospasm. New York : Alan R. Liss, Inc 1986; 1-29.
3. Higgins MW, Lenfant CJM. Trends in Cornary Heart Disease. Arch Mal Cœur 1989; Vol 7, 82 : 2041-7.
4. Sexton RC, Rudney H. Regulation of Cholesterol Biosynthesis. Ann Review Nutr 1986; 6 : 245-272.
5. Dyerberg J., Bang HO. Lipid Metabolism, Atherogenesis, and Haemostasis in Eskimos : The Role of the Prostaglandin-3 Family. Haemostasis 1979; 8 (3-5) : 227-33.
6. Kinsella, JE. Seafoods and Fish Oils in Human Health and Disease. New York : Marcel Dekker, Inc 1987.
7. Bruckner G, Webb P, Greenwell L *et al*. Fish Oil Increases Peripheral Capillary Blood Cell Velocity in Humans. Atherosclerosis 1987; 66 : 237-45.
8. Lands VEM. Fish and Human Health. Orlando : Academic Press 1986.
9. Webb P, Bond V, Kotchen T *et al*. Polyunsaturated Fatty Acids and Eicosanoids. Biloxi : Am Oil Chemists Soc 1987; 329-333.

10. Grundy SM. Comparison of Monounsaturated Fatty Acids and Carbohydrates for Lowering Plasma Cholesterol. NEJM 1986; 314 : 745-48.
11. Schwartz RW, Freedman AM, Richardson DR, *et al.* Capillary Blood Flow : Videodensitometry in the Atherosclerotic Patient. J Vas Surg 1984; 1 : 800-808.
12. Ross R, Glomset J. The Pathogenesis of Atherosclerosis. NEJM 1976; 295 : 369-376.
13. Knapp HR. Ω-3 fatty acids, Endogenous Prostaglandins, and Blood Pressure Regulation in Humans. Nutr Rev 1989; 47 : 301-313.
14. Kobayashi S, Hirai A, Terano T *et al.* Reduction in Blood Viscosity by Eicosapentaenoic Acid. Lancet 1981; 2 : 197.
15. Fisher S, Weber PG. Prostaglandin I3 is Formed *in vivo* in Man after Dietary Eicosapentanaeonoic Acid. Nature 1984; 307 : 165-67.
16. Juan H, Sametz. Vascular Reactivity and High Deietary Eicosapentaenoic Acid. Naunyn-Schmiedeberg's Pharmacol 1986; 24 : 631-639.

3

Effect of chronic exposure to cod liver oil and Ω-3 unsaturated fatty acids on endothelium-dependent relaxations

C. Boulanger, V.B. Schini, H. Shimokawa, Th.F. Lüscher, P.M. Vanhoutte

Department of Research, University Hospital, CH-4031 Basel, Switzerland, and Center for Experimental Therapeutics, Baylor College of Medicine, Houston, TX 77030, USA.

Abstract

The endothelium modulates the reactivity of the underlying vascular smooth muscle by releasing vasoactive substances. Thus, the endothelial cells produce prostacyclin and several endothelium-derived relaxing factors, one of which has been identified as nitric oxide. Endothelium-dependent relaxations are augmented in coronary arteries of pigs fed with cod liver oil or with its major component, eicosapentaenoic acid. This is due to an increased production of non-prostanoid relaxing factors from the intima of the blood vessels. An augmented release of relaxing factors also has been demonstrated with cultured endothelial cells chronically exposed to eicosapentaenoic acid. No increase in the production of endothelium-derived nitric oxide could be detected by activation of the soluble guanylate cyclase of cultured endothelial cells, suggesting that chronic exposure to eicosapentaenoic acid augments the release of the yet non-identified endothelium-derived relaxing factor which differs from nitric oxide. Dietary supplementation wich cod liver oil improves endothelium-dependent relaxations in hypercholesterolemic and atherosclerotic blood vessels : this effect could explain - in part - the beneficial effect of Ω-3 fatty acids on the occurence of cardiovascular diseases.

The endothelium modulates the reactivity of the smooth muscle by releasing different relaxing factors [1, 2]. Among these are (a) prostacyclin, produced during activation of the arachidonic acid cascade; (b) endothelium-derived relaxing factor (EDRF) recently identified as the radical nitric oxide [3, 5]; and (c) a non-identified endothelium-derived hyperpolarizing factor (EDHF) [6, 7] *(Figure 1)*. These three endothelial mediators induce-each to a certain extent - the relaxation of smooth muscle in a numerous variety of blood vessels including those of humans. This brief review will summarize the effect of chronic exposure to cod-liver oil or to Ω-3 unsaturated fatty acid on endothelium-dependent relaxations and the production of non-prostanoid relaxing factors by endothelial cells.

Relaxing factors produced by the endothelium

A non-prostanoid relaxing factor [3] released by the vascular endothelium shares pharmacological properties with the radical nitric oxide [8, 9]. In many bioassay studies, the release of nitric oxide from endothelial cells and from the endothelium of isolated blood vessels accounts for the relaxing activity of the perfusate [4, 10]. As endothelium-derived relaxing factor, nitric oxide induces relaxation of vascular smooth muscle by activating soluble guanylate cyclase and this effect is inhibited by methylene blue; nitric oxide is also scavenged by hemoglobin and inactivated by superoxide anions. Nitric oxide is synthetized in endothelial cells from the amino acid L-arginine [11]. The enzymatic conversion of L-arginine to nitric oxide is inhibited by an L-N^G monomethyl analog of the amino acid [12]. *In vivo* blockade of nitric oxide synthesis leads to an increase in blood pressure [5]. However, the release of nitric oxide from the endothelium as a single radical is still controversial : for example, nitric oxide might bind a carrier, the amino acid cysteine, and be released as nitrocysteine [13].

In addition to nitric oxide, endothelial cells release another relaxing factor, called endothelium-derived hyperpolarizing factor (EDHF). In canine arteries, the relaxation and the hyperpolarization of the smooth muscle that EDHF induces are sensitive to ouabain [6]. Endothelium-derived nitric oxide does not modify the membrane potential of arterial smooth muscle and its effect is insensitive to ouabain [14]. The relaxing factor that differs from nitric oxide has a more pronounced effect in blood vessels of small diameter [15]. Endothelium-derived hyperpolarizing factor could initiate the endothelium-dependent relaxations; alternatively, it could increase the action of nitric oxide on smooth muscle.

Effect of chronic exposure to cod liver oil

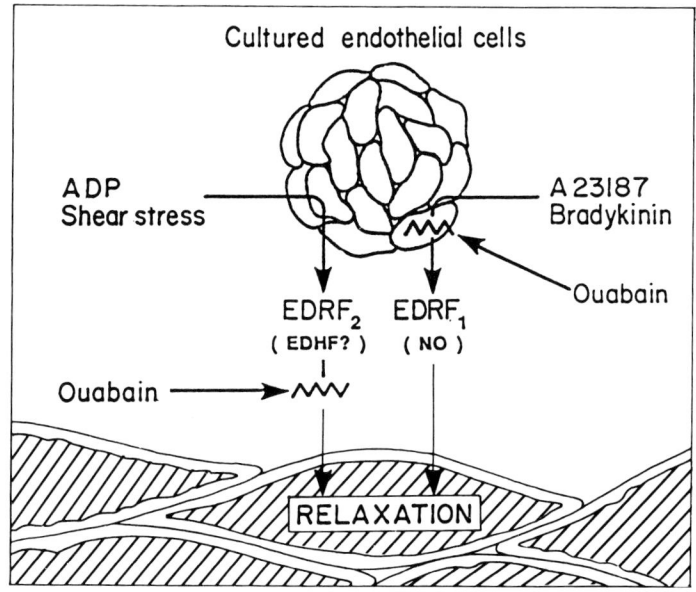

Figure 1. Schematic representation of the release of at least two different relaxing factors from cultured porcine endothelial cells. Bradykinin and the calcium ionophore A23187 release by a ouabain-sensitive mechanism, a relaxing factor which induces relaxation of canine coronary smooth muscle as nitric oxide does. The effect of the relaxing factor released by adenosine diphosphate (ADP) and under shear stress conditions, is impaired in the presence of ouabain; this relaxing factor possesses similar properties to endothelium-derived hyperpolarizing factor (EDHF). (From reference [16], by permission).

The release of prostanoids and non-prostanoids relaxing factors can be observed from cultured endothelial cells. The relaxing activity of the superfusate of cultured endothelial cells grown on microcarrier beads and packed into a chromatographic column is assessed usually using a ring of blood vessel without endothelium as detector. The influence of vasoactive prostanoids can be ruled out by performing the experiments in the presence of an inhibitor of cyclooxygenase. The release of non-prostanoid relaxing factors can be observed both under basal conditions and upon stimulation with bradykinin, adenosine diphosphate or the calcium inophore A23187 *(Figure 1)* [16]. Under these bioassay conditions, cultured endothelial cells from the porcine aorta release two relaxing factors, one being most likely nitric oxide. These two factors can be differentiated with ouabain. Bradykinin and the calcium inophore A23187 release a relaxing factor which is similar to nitric oxide; its action is unopposed by ouabain. Another relaxing factor is released spontaneously or upon stimulation with adenosine diphosphate : its effect on vascular smooth muscle is inhibited by the cardenolide [16]. Methylene blue

33

and hemoglobin inhibit the relaxation induced by exogenous nitric oxide and that induced by bradykinin; however, they only partially impair that mediated by adenosine diphosphate.

Effect of cod-liver oil and Ω-3 unsaturated fatty acids on endothelium-dependent relaxations

Dietary supplementation with cod-liver oil increases the endothelium-dependent relaxations of porcine coronary arteries induced by aggregating platelets, bradykinin, thrombin and products of platelet aggregation, but not those mediated by the calcium ionophore A23187 *(Figure 2)* [17]. This indicates that the basic process leading to the release of endothelium-derived relaxing factor(s) is not affected. The same effect induced by cod-fish oil can be reproduced in large coronary arteries and coronary microvessels of pigs fed with eicosapentaenoic acid, the major component of marine oils [18, 19] *(Figure 3)*. Bioassay experiments demonstrate that bradykinin releases relaxing factors to a greater extent from the intima of blood vessels obtained from animals treated with the Ω-3 unsaturated fatty acid [18].

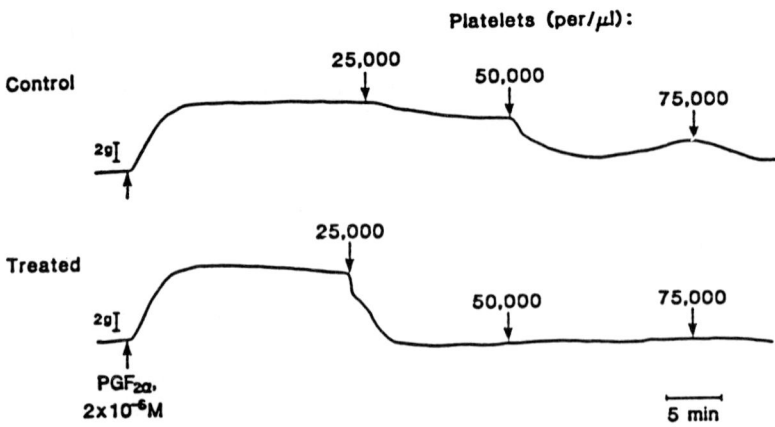

Figure 2. Effect of chronic intake of cod-liver oil on the response of porcine coronary arteries to aggregating platelets. The porcine coronary arteries with endothelium were first contracted with prostaglandin F2alpha (PGF2α) before the addition of increasing number of platelets to the organ chambers. Please note the higher relaxation induced by the platelets in the blood vessels of animals fed with cod liver oil. (From reference [17], by permission).

Effect of chronic exposure to cod liver oil

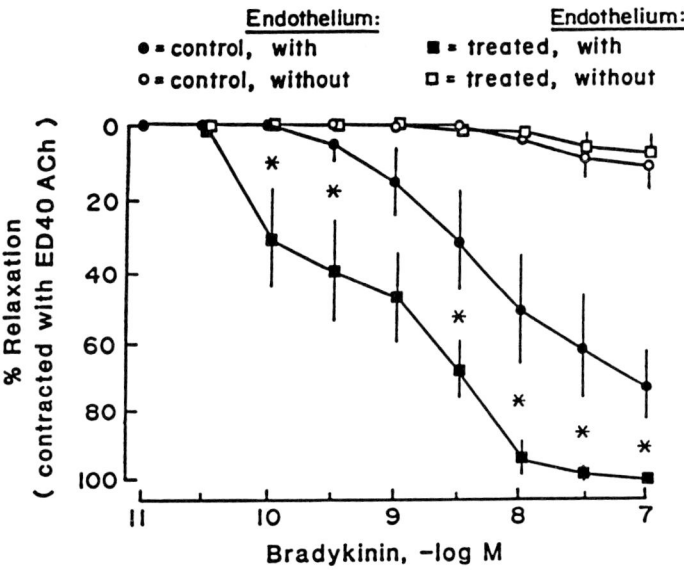

Figure 3. Effect of dietary supplementation of pigs with Ω3-unsaturated fatty acids on the response of porcine coronary resistance microvessels with endothelium to bradykinin. Experiments were realized in the presence of indomethacin to inhibit the production of vasoactive prostanoids. (From Reference [18], with permission).

In order to delineate which of the endothelial mediators was involved in the response induced by chronic exposure to Ω-3 fatty acids, cultured endothelial cells were exposed for several days to eicosapentaenoic acid (2.5×10^{-5} M). The release of relaxing substances from cultured endothelial cells was determined under bioassay conditions [20]. Chronic exposure to eicosapentaenoic acid augmented the relaxations mediated by bradykinin and to a larger extent those induced by adenosine diphosphate, but it did not affect those evoked by the calcium ionophore A23187 *(Figure 4)*. The production of endothelium-derived nitric oxide by cultured endothelial cells can be detected by the activation of the soluble guanylate cyclase and further accumulation of cyclic GMP in the endothelial cells. Stimulation of cultured endothelial cells by exogenous nitric oxide and by agents releasing relaxing factor(s) induced a rapid and transient increase of the intracellular level of cyclic GMP which was inhibited by methylene blue and by L-N^G monomethyl arginine [21]. No difference in cyclic GMP accumulation was found in cells exposed to eicosapentaenoic acid when compared to control *(Figure 5)*. These results suggest that chronic exposure to eicosapentaenoic acid does not improve the production of endothelium-derived nitric oxide but favors the release of another non-prostanoid relaxing factor [20].

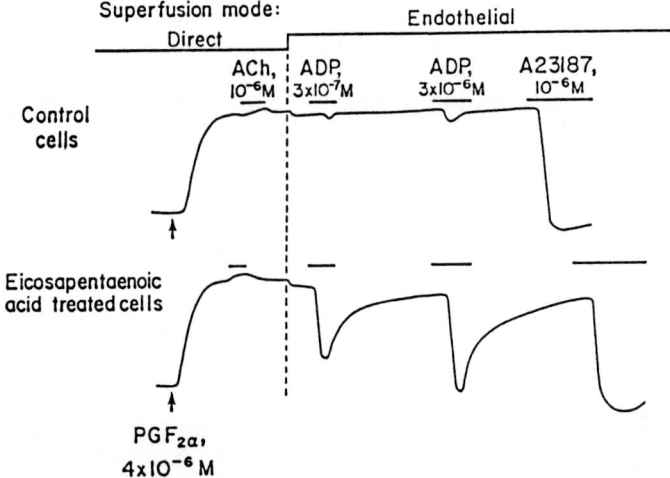

Figure 4. Effect of chronic exposure of cultured endothelial cells to eicosapentaenoic acid on the production of relaxing factors under bioassay condition. The relaxing activity of a perfusate of control or eicosapentaenoic-acid treated endothelial cells was assessed with a canine coronary artery rings (bioassay rings) without endothelium. The bioassay ring were contracted under a column of beads without cells with prostaglandin F2 α, and then moved under a column of microcarrier beads coated with cultured endothelial cells to detect the release of relaxing factors upon stimulation with adenosine diphosphate (ADP) or the calcium ionophore A23187. The relaxing activity of the perfusate from cells exposed to eicopentaenoic acid was higher than that observed with control cultures. (From reference [20], by permission).

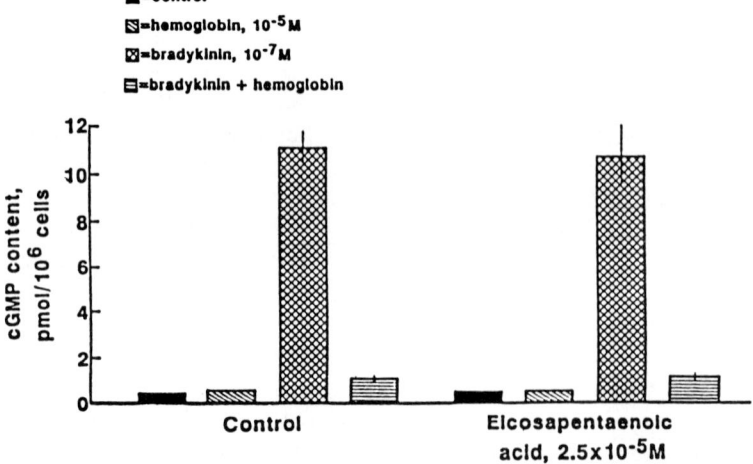

Figure 5. Effect of chronic exposure of cultured endothelial cells to eicosapentaenoic acid on the production of cyclic GMP upon stimulation with bradykinin. The accumulation of cyclic GMP was determined after 1 min stimulation, in the presence of indomethracin and isobutylmethyl xanthine. Cyclic GMP was determined with a radioimmunoassay and expressed as pmol/million cells. (From reference [20], by permission).

Ω-3 unsaturated fatty acids and cardiovascular disease

Dysfunction of the endothelial layer plays a major role in the pathogenesis of atherosclerosis [22]. The endothelium-dependent responses to aggregating platelets and related vasoactive substances (serotonin and adenosine diphosphate) are impaired in coronary arteries of hyper-cholesterolemic pigs or in those with regenerated endothelium [23, 24]. These responses are blunted even further in atherosclerotic blood vessels. This impaired relaxation is probably due to a reduced release of endothelium-derived relaxing factors [23]. The interactions between platelets and atherosclerotic blood vessels would favor platelet aggregation and platelets-induced contractions of vascular smooth muscle; this could lead to vasospasm and thrombosis. Dietary supplementation with Ω-3 unsaturated fatty acids may delay the impairment of endothelium-dependent relaxations in hypercholesterolemia and in atherosclerosis, partly by improving the release of endothelium-derived relaxing factors [25, 26] *(Figure 6)*.

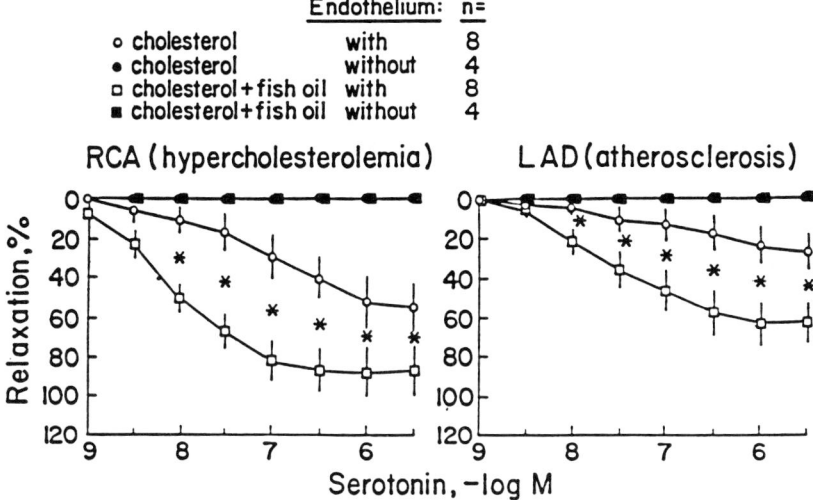

Figure 6. Effect of dietary supplementation with cod liver oil of pigs fed with a regime high in cholesterol on endothelium-dependent relaxation evoked by serotonin in coronary arteries. Compare the response of the right coronary artery (RCA) to that of the left descending coronary artery (LAD), with has been previously denuded by the means of a balloon catheter. Experiments were performed in the presence of indomethacin and ketanserin. (From Reference [25], with permision).

References

1. Furchgott RF, Vanhoutte PM. Endothelium-derived relaxing and contracting factors. The Faseb J 1989; 3 : 2007-2018.
2. Lüscher TF, Vanhoutte PM. The endothelium : Modulator of cardiovascular function. CRC Press, Boca Raton, 1990 (in press).
3. Furchgott RF, Zawadzki JV. The obligatory role of endothelial cells in the relaxation of arterial smooth muscle by acetylcholine. Nature 1980; 299 : 373-376.
4. Palmer RMJ, Ferrige AG, Moncada S. Nitric oxide release accounts for the biological activity of endothelium-derived relaxing factor. Nature 1987; 327 : 524-526.
5. Rees DD, Palmer RMJ, Moncada S. The role of endothelium-derived nitric oxide in the regulation of blood pressure. Proc Natl Acad Sci USA 1989; 86 : 3375-3378.
6. Feletou M, Vanhoutte PM. Endothelium-dependent hyperpolarization of canine coronary smooth muscle. Br J Pharmacol 1988; 93 : 515-524.
7. Bény J-L, Brunet PC. Electrophysiological and mechanical effects of substance P and acetylcholine on rabbit aorta. J Physiol 1988; 398 : 277-289.
8. Furchgott RF, Khan MT, Jothianandan D *et al*. Evidence that the endothelium-derived relaxing factor of rabbit aorta is nitric oxide. *In : Vascular Neuroeffector Mechanisms* Vol 10, Bevan JA, Majewski H, Maxwell RA and Story DF, eds, IRL Press, Oxford, England, 1988; pp 77-84.
9. Ignarro LJ, Byrns RE, Wood KS. Biochemical and pharmacological properties of endothelium-derived relaxing factor and its similarity to nitric oxide radical. *In : Vasodilatation : Vascular Smooth Muscle, Peptides, Autonomic Nerves and Endothelium*. PM Vanhoutte, ed, Raven Press, New York, NY, 1988; pp 427-436.
10. Amezcua JL, Dusting GJ, Palmer RMJ *et al*. Acetylcholine induces vasodilatation in the rabbit isolated heart through the release of nitric oxide, the endogenous nitrovasodilator. Br J Pharmacol 1988; 95 : 830-834.
11. Palmer RMJ, Ashton DS, Moncada S. Vascular endothelial cells synthesize nitric oxide from L-arginine. Nature 1988; 333 : 664-666.
12. Rees DD, Palmer RMJ, Hodson HF *et al*. A specific inhibitor of nitric oxide formation from L-arginine attenuates endothelium-dependent relaxation. Br J Pharmacol 1989; 96 : 418-424.
13. Myers PR, Guerra R Jr, Bates JN *et al*. Studies on the properties of endothelium-derived relaxing factor (EDRF), nitric oxide, and nitrosothiols : Similarities between EDRF and S-nitroso-L-cysteine (cysNO) (Abstract). J Vasc Med Biol 1989; 1/2 : 106.
14. Komori K, Lorenz RR, Vanhoutte PM. Nitric oxide, acetylcholine, and electrical and mechanical properties of canine arterial smooth muscle. Am J Physiol 1988; 255 : H207-H212.
15. Hoeffner U, Boulanger C, Vanhoutte PM. Proximal and distal coronary arteries respond differently to basal EDRF but not to NO. Am J Physiol 1989; 256 : H828-H831.
16. Boulanger C, Hendrickson H, Lorenz RR *et al*. Release of different relaxing factors by cultured porcine endothelial cells. Circ Res 1989; 64 : 1070-1078.

17. Shimokawa H, Lam JYT, Chesebro JH et al. Effects of dietary supplementation with cod-liver oil on endothelium-dependent responses in porcine coronary arteries. Circulation 1987; 76 : 898-905.
18. Shimokawa H, Aarhus LL, Vanhoutte PM. Dietary Ω-3 polyunsaturated fatty acids augment endothelium-dependent relaxation to bradykinin in porcine coronary microvessels. Br J Pharmacol 1989; 95 : 1191-1196.
19. Shimokawa H, Vanhoutte PM. Dietary Ω-3 fatty acids and endothelium-dependent relaxations in porcine coronary arteries. Am J Physiol 1989; 256 : H968-H973.
20. Boulanger C, Schini VB, Hendrickson H et al. Chronic exposure of cultured endothelial cells to eicosapentaenoic acid potentiates the release of endothelium-derived relaxing factor(s). Br J Pharmacol 1990; 99 : 176-180.
21. Boulanger C, Schini VB, Vanhoutte PM. Production of cyclic GMP by bradykinin, adenosine diphosphate, the calcium ionophore A23187 and nitric oxide in cultured porcine aortic endothelial cells. Faseb J 1989; 3 : A533.
22. Ross R. The pathogenesis of atherosclerosis- An update. New Engl J Med 1986; 314 : 488-500.
23. Shimokawa H, Vanhoutte PM. Impaired endothelium-dependent relaxation to aggregating platelets and related vasoactive substances in porcine coronary arteries in hypercholesterolemia and atherosclerosis. Circ Res 1989; 64 : 900-914.
24. Shimokawa H, Aarhus LL, Vanhoutte PM. Porcine coronary arteries with regenerated endothelium have a reduced endothelium-dependent responsiveness to aggregating platelets and serotonin. Circ Res 1987; 61 : 256-270.
25. Shimokawa H, Vanhoutte PM. Dietary cod-liver oil improves endothelium-dependent responses in hypercholesterolemic and atherosclerotic porcine coronary arteries. Circulation 1988; 78 : 1421-1430.
26. Shimokawa H, Vanhoutte PM. Hypercholesterolemia causes generalized impairment of endothelium-dependent relaxation to aggregating platelets in porcine arteries. J Amer Coll Cardiol 1989; in press.

4

Interaction between Ω-3 fatty acid and platelet phospholipids

M. Lagarde, M. Groset, M. Hajarine

INSERM U205, Chimie biologique INSA, Bât. 406, 69621 Villeurbanne, France.

Abstract

Ω-3 fatty acids, ingested from fish fat, have been recognized as potential inhibitors of some processes involved in atherogenesis and thrombogenesis. Among these, platelet hyperactivity may be efficiently reduced by the two main Ω-3 fatty acids of fish oil, namely eicosapentaenoic (Epa, 20:5 Ω-3) and docosahexaenoic (DHA, 22:6 Ω-3) acids, both *in vivo* and *in vitro*. Most of this inhibitory activity has been however attributed to EPA, although DHA is generally ingested in similar amounts and some studies have shown the efficacy of pure DHA intake. We report *in vitro* studies comparing platelet enrichment with EPA or DHA, revealing that DHA is rather more potent than EPA in inhiting platelet aggregation. Their mechanism of action differs entirely, especially at the phospholipid level. Whereas EPA is released from phospholipid subclasses similarly to endogenous arachidonic acid, and competes for the formation of thromboxane A_2, DHA not released virtually but efficiently transferred from phosphatidylcholine to phosphatidylenolamine during platelet activation. Concomitantly to this peculiar phospholipid metabolism, DHA also decreases thromboxane formation from endogenous arachidonic acid and thromboxane-induced aggregation as well as its specific binding to platelet membranes.

We conclude that an original metabolism of DHA at the membrane phospholipid level could explain most of its biological activity in platelets.

Introduction

Since the epidemiological studies by Dyeberg *et al.* [1] showing a very low frequency of cardiovascular diseases in Eskimos, number of investigations have confirmed the potential protective effect of fish fat against atherosclerosis and thrombosis [2]. This may be due to beneficial effects on plasma lipoproteins [3] as well as on blood and vascular cells involved in these pathological processes [4].

Among these cells, platelets and endothelial cells have been well investigated. One feature concerns the inhibition of thromboxane A_2 formation form platelet arachidonic acid (AA) by EPA [5] while the latter is converted into thromboxane A_3 devoid of pro-aggregatory and vasoconstrictor properties [6]. In contrast, the vascular endothelium converts EPA into prostaglandin I_3 which shares the biological activity of prostaglandin I_2 (prostacyclin) [7]. It is then assumed that overall, the balance between thromboxane and prostacyclin is shifted towards its anti-aggregatory and vasodilating potential, which could explain the beneficial effect of fish fat intakes in preventing atherosclerosis and thrombosis.

EPA is also believed to reduce the activity of blood cells involved in inflammation which might contribute in these pathological processes. This refers in particular to leukocytes and their production of leukotriene B_4, a potent chemotactic agent, and of platelet-activating factor (PAF), a pro-inflammatory phospholipid acting at several stages of the inflammatory process. Leukotriene B_4 production is decreased and partially replaced by leukotriene B5 which is much less active than its analogue B_4 [8], while PAF generation is markedly reduced [9].

Although DHA is consumed in similar amount as EPA in various fish fat preparations, few investigations have been performed to precise its contribution in the effects observed [10]. These investigations concern mainly platelets and reveal that DHA could be even more potent than EPA in preventing platelet aggregation [11, 12].

We report here that the mechanism of action for platelet inhibition by DHA differs entirely from that of EPA, with special reference to platelet phospholipid metabolism.

Phospholipid metabolism

When studied *in vitro* via the Lands pathway (acylation/deacylation) [13], EPA and DHA, pre-coated onto albumin, are efficiently taken up by human platelets. The main unesterified polyunsaturated fatty acid of the normal human plasma, linoleic acid (LA) and AA, are able to compete with the uptake of EPA and DHA. The study was done in the presence of ten fold higher concentration of LA and equal concentration of AA to simulate the physiological ratio between these latter fatty acids in plasma. Although both LA and AA reduced the total incorporation of EPA and DHA into platelet lipid pools. AA proved to be more active than LA, suggesting that the closest configuration off AA, compared to EPA and DHA, is crucial for competing at the uptake stage. Under the above mentioned conditions, 90 % of EPA and 80 % of DHA are acylated in glycerophospholipids, the remaining being acylated in neutral lipids, mainly triacyglycerols, especially for DHA [14]. Looking at the glycerophospholipid class distribution of each of both EPA and DHA, we found a substantial difference in which EPA was mainly acylated into phosphatidylcholine (PC) (> 60 %) with only 10 % in phosphalidylethanolamine (PE) whereas DHA was distributed according to 40 and 30 %, respectively. This agrees with the general assumption that DHA is preferentially located in PE of most tissues [15].

In the presence of aggregating agents inducing platelet phospholipase activities like thrombin and the calcium ionophore A23187, EPA is released from total phospholipids but DHA is not. The percentage release of EPA is quite similar to that of AA from its endogenous pool. At the level of each glycerophospholipid, a very marked difference could be observed between both Ω-3 fatty acid. EPA behaves quite similarly as endogenous AA with a release from PC and secondarily from phosphatidylinositol (PI). The release from PI might be not relevant since the incorporation of EPA into PI appears to be very low *in vivo* [16]. Unexpectingly, DHA is released markedly from PC and reacylated reciprocally into PE [17]. The reciprocal reacylation of DHA into PE is likely to explain the absence of release observed when examined at the total glycerophospholipid level.

Oxygenated metabolism

Subsequently to its release from membrane phospholipids, EPA is efficiently oxygenated via the 12-lipoxygenase pathway, and to a lesser entent via the cyclooxygenase/thromboxane synthase pathway [18]. The efficient oxygenation can occur because of the simultaneous released AA which is concomitantly converted into its lipoxygenase product, 12-hydroperoxyeicosatetraenoic acid [12-HPETE]. This peroxyde potentiates very markedly the oxygenation of EPA [19, 20]. In addition to the reduced thromboxane

A_2 formation, the production of substantial amount of the end-lipoxygenase product of EPA (12-HEPE) could contribute to platelet inhibition in antagonizing thromboxane A_2 – induced platelet aggregation [21, 22].

In contrast, DHA virtually is not oxygenated, although its convertion by platelet lipoxygenase is also potentiated efficiently by AA, presumably via 12-HPETE [23]. This is likely due to the absence of its release from membrane phospholipids and suggests, that the marked transfer observed from PC to PE under platelet stimulation occurs without substantial liberation.

Simultaneously the oxygenation of endogenous AA into prostanoids is decreased in EPA- or DHA-rich platelets while the lipoxygenation of AA is not altered [23]. The cyclooxygenase and thromboxane synthase being membrane bound enzymes whereas the lipoxygenase is cytosolic, this may indicate that EPA and DHA might inhibit the enzyme at the level of membrane lipid-protein interactions.

Conclusion

From these results we may conclude that the two main polyunsaturated fatty acids from fish fat are both efficient inhibitors of platelet function *in vitro*, but act through entirely different mechanism. Whereas EPA competes with the endogenous AA at several stages, DHA prevents platelet aggregation by different ways, among these the specific transfer between PC and PE could be important to account for.

References

1. Dyeberg J, Bang HO, Stoffersen E *et al*. Eicosapentaenoic acid and prevention of thrombosis and atherosclerosis. Lancet 1978; ii : 117-19.
2. Leaf A and Weber PC. Cardiovascular effects of n-3 fatty acids. New Engl J Med 1988; 318 : 549-57.
3. Goodnight SH, Harris SH, Connor WE *et al*. Polyunsaturated fatty acids, hyperlipidemia and thrombosis. Artheriosclerosis 1982; 2 : 87-113.
4. Ross R. The pathogenesis of atherosclerosis – an update. New Engl J Med 1986; 314 : 488-500.
5. Siess W, Roth P, Scherer B *et al*. Platelet membrane fatty acids, platelet aggregation, and thromboxane formation during a mackerel diet. Lancet 1980; i : 441-4.

6. Needleman Ph, Raz A, Minkes Ms et al. Triene prostaglandins : prostacyclin and thromboxane biosynthesis. A unique biological properties. Proc Natl Sci USA 1979; 76 : 744-8.
7. Fisher S, Weber PC, Prostaglandin I₃ is formed *in vivo* in man after dietary eicosapentaenoic acid. Nature 1984; 307 : 165-8.
8. Terano T, Salmon JA, Moncada S. Biosynthesis and biological activity of leukotriene B₅. Protaglandins 1984; 27 : 217-32.
9. Pickett WE, Nytko D, Dondero-Zahn C et al. The effect of endogenous eicosapentaenoic acid on PMN leukotriène and PAF biosynthesis. Prostagland Leuk Med 1986; 23 : 135-40.
10. Lagarde M. Metabolism of fatty acids by platelets and the function of various metabolites in mediating platelet function. Progr Lipid Res 1988; 27 : 135-52.
11. V Schacky C, Weber PC. Metabolism and effect on platelet function of the purified eicosapentaenoic and docosahexaenoid acids in humans. J Clin Invest 1985; 76 : 2446-50.
12. Croset M, Lagarde M. *In vitro* incorporation and metabolism of eicosapentaenoic and docosahexaenoic acids in human platelets. Effect on aggregation. Throm Haemost 1986; 56 : 57-62.
13. Lands Wem, Heart P. Control of fatty acid composition in glycerol phospholipids J Am Oil Chem Soc 1965; 43 : 290-5.
14. Hajarine M, Lagarde M. Studies on polyenoic acid incorporation into human platelet lipid stores : interactions with linoleic and arachidonic acids. Biochim Biophys Acta 1986; 877 : 299-304.
15. Tinoco. Dietary requirements and functions of α-linolenic acid in animals. Progr Lipid Res 1982; 21 : 1-45.
16. Galloway JH, Cortwright IJ, Woodcock BE et al. Effects of dietary fish oil supplementation on the fatty acid composition of human platelet membrane : demonstration of selectivity in the incorporation of eicosapentaenoic acid into membrane phospholipids. Clin Sci 1985; 68 : 449-54.
17. Hajarine M, Lagarde M. Liberation and oxygenation of polyenoic acids in stimulated platelets. Biochimic 1988; 70 : 1749-58.
18. Lagarde M, Drouot B, Guichardant M et al. *In vitro* incorporation and metabolism of some eicosaenoic acids in platelets. Effect on arachidonic acid oxygenation. Biochim Biophys Acta 1985; 833 : 52-8.
19. Morita I, Takahashi R, Saito Y et al. Stimulation of eicosapentaenoic acid metabolism in washed human platelets by 12-hydroperoxy-eicosatetraenoic acid. J Biol Chem 1983; 258 : 10297-99.
20. Croset M, Lagarde M. Enhancement of eicosaenoic acid lipoxygenation in human platelets by 12-hydroperoxy derivative of arachidonic acid. Lipids 1985; 20 : 743-50.
21. Croset M, Lagarde M. Stereospecific inhibition of PGH$_2$-induced platelet aggregation by lipoxygenase products of icosaenoic acids. Biochem Biophys Res Commun 1983; 112 ; 879-83.
22. Coene MC, Bult H, Claeys M et al. Inhibition of rabbit platelet activation by lipoxygenase products of arachidonic and linoleic acids. Thromb Res 1986; 42 : 205-14.
23. Croset M, Guichardant M, Lagard M. Different metabolic behavior of long chain Ω-3 polyunsaturated fatty acids in human platelets. Biochim Biophys Acta 1988; 961 : 262-9.

5

Pharmacological modulation of venular permeability with some antiinflammatory drugs

E. Svensjö

Department of Exploratory Pharmacology, Draco, Lund, Sweden

Introduction

Endothelial cells in culture respond to histamine and bradykinin stimulation with an immediate rise in intracellular concentration of Ca and inositolphosphates [1-4].
The functional response to receptor-mediated stimulation of endothelial cells *in vitro* could be demonstrated by measuring the passage of a macromolecular tracer (albumin) through widened cell junctions. In the same study it was also shown that histamine induced cytoskeletal changes in terms of a reduced F-actin content which is a sign of actin polymerisation and cellular contraction resulting in widened junctions or gaps [1].
These recent studies support the original proposal by Majno and Palade [5] that endothelial cells in postcapillary venules could contract on stimulation with serotonin and histamine. They demonstrated the escape of carbon particles, and by implication plasma leakage, from the vasculature at the level of postcapillary venules. The site of plasma leakage in the microvasculature has also been shown by combining intravital and electron microscopy of the same vascular bed [6]. Fluorescein labeled dextran (FITC-dextran,

MW=150,000) was given i.v. to hamsters and the cheek pouch microvasculature was observed by intravital microscopy. Extravasation of FITC-dextran (plasma leakage) was only observed in postcapillary venules after stimulation with bradykinin. The leaking venules were subjected to electron microscopy which could show electron dense precipitates of FITC-dextran in the vessel lumen, in the widened junctions (gaps) of postcapillary venules and in the interstitium [6].

The described technique of visualizing plasma leakage by intravital microscopy can show increased vascular permeability due to direct endothelial stimulation at the earliest 30 seconds after mediator application and will reach a maximum response at 3-5 min [7]. However, electrophysiological measurements of resistance of the endothelial cell lining in capillaries *in vivo* have shown that serotonin stimulation could reduce resistance within a second reaching a minimum within 10 seconds which is in analogy with the immediate response seen in cultured endothelial cells [8]. Measurements of nonstimulated arterioles and venules showed that there was a lower resistance on the venous side providing further evidence to why these vessels are more prone to leak [9]. Morphological studies have shown that a certain fraction, 25-30 %, of the intercellular junctions in postcapillary venules is open to a gap already under nonstimulated conditions [10].

The gathered view from *in vitro* and *in vivo* studies of endothelial cell functions supports the hypothesis that a physiological and pharmacological regulation of macromolecular permeability is exerted by the endothelial cells in the postcapillary venules [11-14]. This report will briefly describe the technique for vascular permeability studies in the cheek pouch preparation and give some results from studies on how the action of several inflammatory mediators could be modified by different pharmacological principles which probably act directly on the endothelial cells.

Material and methods

The use of the hamster cheek pouch for studies of macromolecular permeability has been described [7, 15, 16]. For microscopic observations the single layer cheek pouch preparation is performed essentially as described by Duling [17] with our modifications [16].

The hamster is anesthetized with pentobarbital and the cheek pouch is gently everted and mounted on the microscopic stage. The pouch is submerged in a pool and continuously superfused with a bicarbonate buffered saline solution

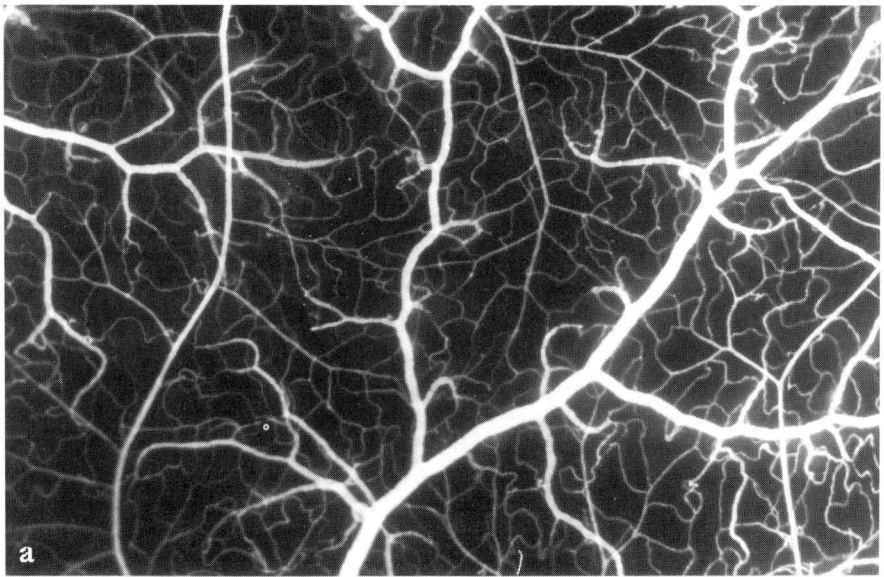

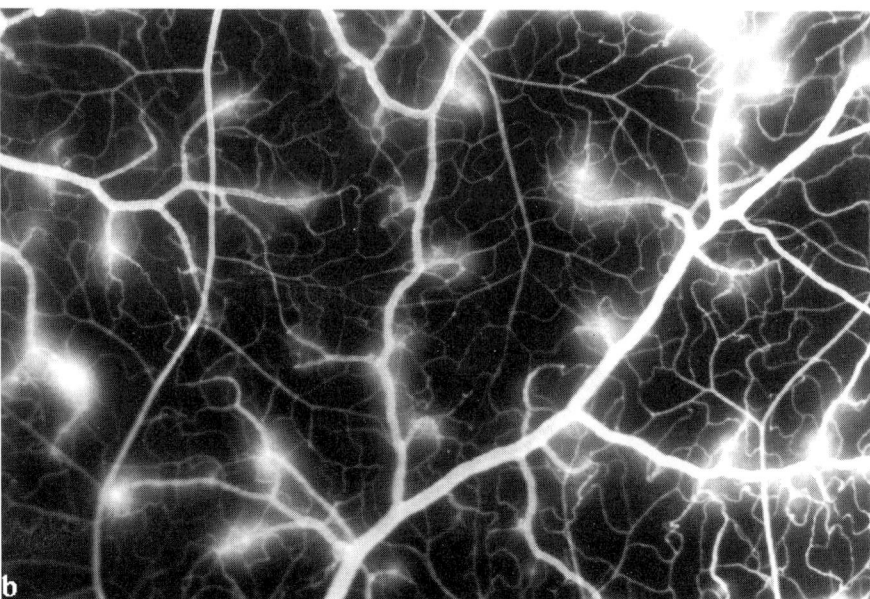

Figure 1. – Fluorescent micrograph of the hamster cheek pouch after i.v. injection of 150,000-dalton FITC-dextran. Same area before (a) and 5 min after (b) topical application of bradykinin 4×10^{-7} M for 5 min. Several leakage sites at postcapillary venules are shown by extravasation of FITC-dextran.

at a constant flow. The superfusion solution is fed into a cuvette of a fluorimeter for continuous measurements of FITC-dextran concentration. Properly dissected the hamster cheek pouch preparation gives excellent optical resolution and is an untraumatized preparation to judge from the presence of vascular tone (vasomotion) and the absence of FITC-dextran leakage sites or intravascular leukocyte accumulation for several hours.

Illumination of the preparation with a 100 W Hg lamp and filtering of the light for FITC-microscopy clearly reveal the intravascular FITC-dextran *(Figure 1 a)* and how FITC-dextran is leaking from postcapillary venules following topical application of bradykinin *(Figure 1 b)*.

In most preparations there is no visible extravasation of FITC-dextran (leakage sites) although the concentration of FITC-dextran in the superfusing buffer increases immediately (in less than 3 min) after its injection to reach a maximum around 30 minutes later. Preparations with no or fading leaks and no further increase in FITC-dextran concentration after 30 min are acceptable for experiments [18].

Autacoids and drugs that could affect macromolecular permeability can now be added to the superfusion buffer before it flows over the cheek pouch *(Table I)*. Microvascular leakage is quantitated by counting the number of leaks per cm^2 of the preparation *(Figure 1 b)*. A linear dose-response-rela-

Table I. – Mediators that increase FITC-dextran leakage in postcapillary venules (intravital microscopy)

Mediator	Effective conc., M
Histamine, serotonin	10^{-6}
Bradykinin, substance P	10^{-7}
ADP, adenosine, inosine	10^{-5}
Prostaglandins E_1, E_2, $F_{2\alpha}$	$>10^{-8}$
Leukotrienes C_4, D_4, E_4, B_4	$>10^{-9}$
Complement, C3a, C5a	$>10^{-9}$
Platelet activating factor (PAF)	$>10^{-9}$
Fibrin derived peptides	-
Free radicals, ischemia	-
Immune aggregates	-
Phorbol ester (PDBu)	10^{-6}
Oxidant injury (tertiar-butyl-hydroperoxid)	$4 \cdot 10^{-4}$
Endotoxin (E. coli 0111.B4)	(0.7 µg/ml)

tionship between the number of leaks and the logaritmic dose of bradykinin has been shown [7]. Several leukotrienes (LTC_4, LTD_4, LTA_4, LTB_4) and histamine also induce a linear dose-dependent increase in number of leaks [19]. The number of leaks per cm^2 correlated with the amount of FITC-dextran eliminated by the superfusing buffer during 30 min after stimulation with histamine [18] or LTB_4 [20]. All mediators or noxious agents tested so far *(Table I)* induced a reversible increase in the number of leaks and FITC-dextran concentration of the superfusate as exemplified for LTB_4 *(Figure 2)*.

Modulation of mediator-induced permeability increase

Pharmacological inhibition of mediator-induced leak formation was first shown with a β_2-receptor agonist, terbutaline (0.5mg/kg b.w.), which reduced the bradykinin response by 83 % (21). Since then the inhibitory effect of β_2-agonist has been further characterized by the use of several other mediators [12, 18, 22] listed in *Table II*. The selective β_2-receptor antagonist ICI 118 551 could effectively block the antipermeability effect of terbutaline [22]. The β_2-blocker potentiated the histamine response by 20 % suggesting that endothelial cells may be under some influence of endogenous catecholamines. The specificity of β_2-receptors in postcapillary venules was shown in experiments with the (-)- and (+)-forms of terbutaline given either locally or as i.v. injection. The (+)-form had no effect at concentrations or i.v. doses which were 100 times higher than the effective concentrations or i.v. doses of the (-)-form [22]. The selective inhibition of the mediator-induced permeability increase with the (-)-form has also been shown in the canine forelimb preparation [23].

Several clinically important glucocorticoids, e.g. budesonide, dexamethasone and methylprednisolone (MP), have been studied in the cheek pouch both on local administration and after i.v. injection. Local treatment with the glucocorticoids resulted in a 90 % reduction of the number of histamine-induced leaks, when the glucocorticoid treatment was given 60 min before the histamine challenge [24]. The effect had a slower onset compared with the effects seen with other anti-inflammatory drugs which suggests that glucocorticoids acted on endothelial hormonal receptor, nuclear uptake and release or synthesis of active proteins. Results on immunoaggregate-induced release of histamine also suggested that the anti-permeability effect of MP was induced through a direct action on the endothelium. This release was not affected by MP given 24 hours before ovalbumin challenge. However, MP-treated

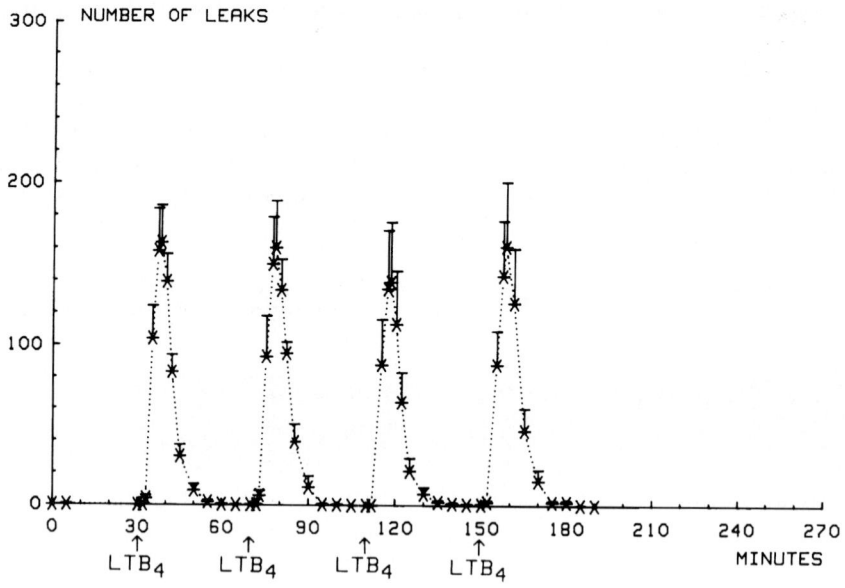

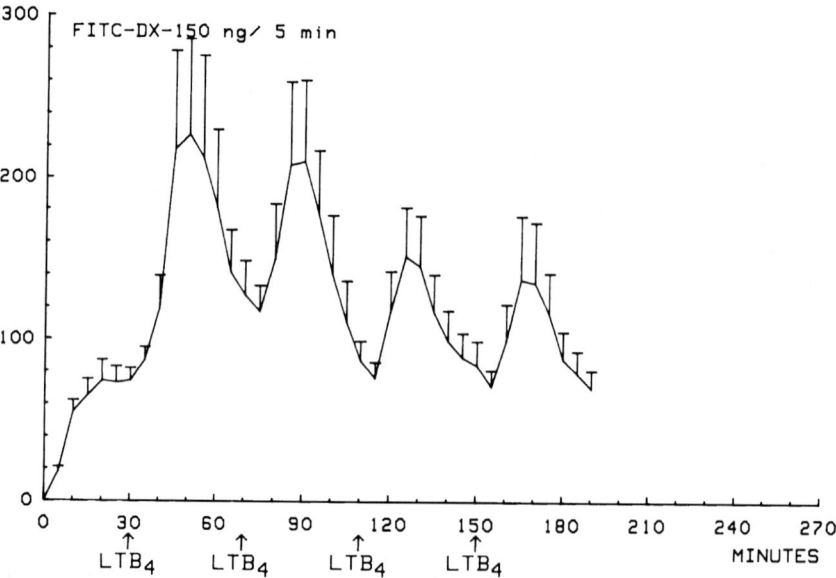

Figure 2. – The permeability increase in the number of leaks (top) and efflux of FITC-dextran (bottom) following four local applications of LTB_4 (10^{-8} M, 5 min) in 6 hamsters (mean ± SEM).

Table II. – Inhibitors of mediator-induced leakage of large molecules (FITC-dextran) in the hamster.

Inhibitor	Conc. M	Mediator
β_2-receptor agonist (terbutaline)	10^{-7}-10^{-6}	Histamine, bradykinin, ischemia, LTB_4 adenosine, phorbol ester, oxidant injury
Calcium antagonist (verapamil)	10^{-5}	Histamine, bradykinin
Glucocorticoids (budesonide, methyl-prednisolon, dexamethason)	10^{-7} (for 5 min) (10 mg/kg iv)	Histamine, bradykinin, LTB_4, LTC_4, PAF, immune agregate, ischemia, oxidant injury, phorbol ester, endotoxin
Theophylline	10^{-5}	Histamine
Vasopressin (and derivatives)	10^{-8}	Bradykinin, histamine
H_1-receptor antagonist (mepyramine)	10^{-5}	Histamine
$5HT_2$-receptor antagonist (ketanserin)	$5 \cdot 10^{-7}$	Serotonin, histamine
PKC-inhibitors H-7, staurosporin	10^{-5}-10^{-8}	Phorbol ester (Phorbol-12-13-dibutyrate, PDBu)
Superoxiddismutase (CuZn-SOD, EC-SOD)	(25 mg/kg iv)	Ischemia, oxidant injury

hamsters showed a reduced response to locally applied LTC_4, histamine and PAF-acether [25].

The fact that only 5 min of exposure was necessary for the glucocorticoids to exert a pronounced effect supports the hypothesis of a local effect on the endothelial cells in the postcapillary venules. As summarized in *Table II* such a short treatment effectively inhibits the action of several chemical mediators including endotoxin. However, the endotoxin-induced adhesion of leukocytes in the post-capillary venules was not reduced by budesonide, only the increase in vascular permeability was inhibited [26].

Phorbol ester (phorbol-12,13-dibutyrate = PDBu) is a potent stimulator of protein kinase C (PKC) and it induced leakage in postcapillary venules but unlike most other mediators *(Table I)* a marked tachyphylaxis was seen at a second PDBu-challenge several hours after the first [27]. Bradykinin stimulation after the two PDBu-applications gave a permeability increase within the normal range. Terbutaline and budesonide inhibited both PDBu and the bradykinin induced plasma leakage. Two putative PKC-inhibitors H-7 (an isoquinolinsulfonamid) and staurosporin inhibited the PDB_U but not the bradykinin induced response thus indicating a more selective inhibitory action than the β_2-receptor agonist and the glucocorticoid [27].

Conclusion

Some examples of pharmacological inhibition of mediator induced venular permeability (plasma leakage) have been presented. The mechanisms behind these antipermeability effects have to be different but at the present state of knowledge they might be explained as a result of direct actions on venular endothelial cells possibly involving relaxation of mediator-contracted endothelial cells.

References

1. Rotrosen D, Gallin JI. Histamine type I receptor occupancy increases endothelial cytosolic calcium, reduces F-actin, and promotes albumin diffusion across cultured endothelial monolayers. J Cell Biol 1986; 103 : 2379-2387.
2. Derian CK, Moskowitz MA. Polyphosphoinositide hydrolysis in endothelial cells and carotid artery segments. J Biol Chem 1986; 261 : 3831-3837.
3. Lambert TL, Kent RS, Whorton AR. Bradykinin stimulation of inositol polyphosphate production in porcine aortic endothelial cells. J Biol Chem 1986; 261 : 15288-15293.
4. Colden-Stanfield M, Schilling WP, Ritchie AK, *et al.* Bradykinin-induced increases in cytosolic calcium and ionic currents in cultured bovine aortic endothelial cells. Circ Rest 1987; 61 : 632-640.
5. Majno G, Palade GE. Studies on inflammation. I. The effect of histamine and serotonin on vascular permeability. An electron microscopic study. J Biophys Biochem Cytol 1961 ; 11 : 571.
6. Hultström D, Svensjö E. Intravital and electron microscopic study of bradykinin-induced vascular permeability changes using FITC-dextran as a tracer. J Pathol 1979, 129 : 125.
7. Svensjö E. Bradykinin and prostaglandin E_1, E_2 and $F_{2\alpha}$-induced macromolecular leakage in the hamster cheek pouch. Prostaglandines and Medicine 1978; 1 : 397-410.
8. Olesen S-P, Crone C. Substances that rapidly augment ionic conductance of endothelium in cerebral venules. Acta Physiol Scand 1986; 127 : 233-241.
9. Olesen S-P. Electrical resistance of arterioles and venules in the hamster cheek pouch. 1985; 123 : 121-126.
10. Simionescu N, Simionescu M, Palade GE. Open junctions in the endothelium of the postcapillary venules of the diaphragm. J Cell Biol 1978; 79 : 27.
11. Grega GJ, Svensjö E, Haddy FJ. Macromolecular permeability of the microvascular membrane : physiological and pharmacological regulation. Microcirculation 1981; 1 : 325-341.
12. Persson CGA, Svensjö E. Vascular responses and their suppression : drugs interfering with venular permeability. *In : Handbook of inflammation, Vol. 5, The pharmacology of inflammation.* Bonta IL, Bray MA, Parnham MJ, Eds, 1985, Amsterdam, Elsevier, pp 61-82.

13. Svensjö E, Grega GJ. Evidence for endothelial cell-mediated regulation of macromolecular permeability by postcapillary venules. Fed Proc 1986; 45 : 89-95.
14. Crone C. Modulation of solute permeability in microvascular endothelium. Federation Proc 1986; 45 : 77-83.
15. Svensjö E, Arfors K-E, Arturson G, *et al*. The hamster cheek pouch preparation as a model for studies of macromolecular permeability of the microvasculature. Uppsala J Med Sci 1978; 83 : 71-79.
16. Björk J, Smedegård G, Svensjö E, *et al*. The use of the hamster cheek pouch for intravital microscopy studies of microvascular events. Prog Appl Microcirc 1984; 6 : 41-53 (Karger, Basel).
17. Duling BR. The preparation and use of the hamster cheek pouch for studies of the microcirculation. Microvasc Res 1973; 5 : 423-429.
18. Svensjö E, Roempke K. Microvascular aspects on edema formation and its inhibition by β_2-receptor stimulants and some other antiinflammatory drugs. *In : Progress in Microcirculation research II* (CPME, Kensington, Australia), Garlick DG, Perry MA, Courtice FC, Eds, 1985.
19. Bjork J, Arfors KE, Dahlen SE, *et al*. Effects of leukotrienes on vascular permeability and leukocyte adhesion. 1981, *In : " The inflammatory process "*. P Venge and A Lindbom Eds, p. 103-112, Almqvist & Wiksell, Uppsala, Sweden.
20. Erlansson M, Svensjo E, Bergqvist D. Leukotriene B4-induced permeability increase in postcapillary venules and its inhibition by three different antiinflammatory drugs. Inflammation 1989; 13 : 693-705.
21. Svensjö E, Persson CGA, Rutili G. Inhibition of bradykinin induced macromolecular leakage from postcapillary venules by a β2-adrenoceptor stimulant, terbutaline. Acta Physiol Scandl 1977; 101 : 504-506.
22. Svensjö E, Roempke K. Dose-related antipermeability effect of terbutaline and its inhibition by a selective β_2-receptor blocking agent. Agents and Actions 1985; 16 : (1/2), 19-20.
23. Dobbins DE, Buehn MJ, Dabney JM. Bradykinin-mediated edema formation is blocked by levorotatory but not dextrorotatory terbutaline. Microcirc Endoth Lymphatics 1988; 5 : 377-397.
24. Svensjö E, Roempke K. Time-dependent inhibition of bradykinin-induced microvascular permeability increase by local glucocorticoid treatment. Respiration 1984; 46 : (Suppl. 1), 60.
25. Bjork J, Goldschmidt T, Smedegard G, *et al*. Methylprednisolone acts at the endothelial cell level reducing inflammatory responses. Acta Physiol Scand 1985, 123 : 221-224.
26. Svensjö E, Erlansson M, Van den Bos GC. Endotoxininduced increase in leukocyte adherence and macromolecular permeability of postcapillary venules. Agents and Actions 1990; 29 : 21-23.
27. Svensjö E, Roempke K. Inhibition of phorbol ester induced microvascular leakage by a putative protein kinase C inhibitor, terbutaline and budesonide. Int J Microcirc 1988; 7 : p. 85 (abstract).

6

Hemorheological concepts in venous insufficiency and implications for treatment with *Ruscus* extract*

C. Le Devehat, T. Khodabandehlou, M. Vimeux, G. Bondoux

Unité de Recherches d'Hémorhéologie clinique, Centre Hospitalier de Nevers, Centre de Diabétologie, 58320 Pougues-les-Eaux, France

Introduction

The disturbances in rheological properties of the blood are of interest as a possible pathological mechanism of venous stasis and thrombosis. Also of clinical importance is the possibility of hemorheologically oriented treatment of venous insufficiency. The albumin/fibrinogen ratio not only largely determines the viscosity of the plasma, but also affects the whole blood viscosity at low shear rates as the principal factor causing red cell aggregation. In contrast, red cell aggregability is thought to be the principal reason for the increased viscosity of the whole blood at low flow rates. The microrheological changes would thus be both a consequence and a cause of the venous stasis on the post capillary venular compartment. When there is a venous stasis, the red cell aggregates persist because the prevailing local flow forces are

---

*Cyclo-3 Fort

not adequate for their fluid dynamic dispersal. In venous stasis, blood is characterized by disturbances of thixotropy or structural viscosity, that is the increase in viscosity due to retarded flow. Drugs' action upon the red cell aggregation are to be considered as additional useful treatment in patients with venous insufficiency. Thus, in order to explain and confirm the clinical interest of *Ruscus* extract as a treatment for venous insufficiency, a preliminary study in a double blind test with placebo was carried out on 25 patients with venous insufficiency of the lower limbs with varicose.

State of art in microcirculation

The microrheological parameters that determine blood viscosity have an important physiological and physiopathological contribution to the understanding and the treatment of vascular pathologies. Venous pathology is characterized by a relative incapacity of the venous system to return back to the heart. Even if valvular incompetence is its basic etiology, numerous studies have shown that the phenomenon of venous insufficiency also is the result of modifications to the vascular wall and especially of important disturbances in the rheological properties of the blood [1]. The essential characteristic of blood viscosity is its increase in vascular sites where the flow is slowed down. In the veins, in the physiological state, the shear rates are the lowest and stasis phenomena can carry very important hyperpressures. Equally, with veins, the shear stress threshold is more elevated, all the more that the blood circulation is stationary. The microrheological parameters play a determining role in the phenomena of cellular activation and aggregation and also in the appearance of a local ischemia or thrombosis. In venous stasis, the venous blood flow is characterized by an increase in viscosity [2]. If, in vascular sites with high blood flow or high shear rates, the deformability of red cells is the determinant of blood viscosity, in contrast, in vascular sites with low flow or low shear rates, blood viscosity is primarily dependent on the aggregation-disaggregation phenomenon of red cells. These two phenomena of aggregation-disaggregation and of deformability of red cells are the microrheological factors controlling the fundamental processes in hemorheology [3, 4]. The degree of deformation of the red cell depends on exterior forces that act on this red cell and on its intrinsic rheological properties. Since the studies of Fahreus in 1921 on erythrocyte aggregates known as "rouleaux", we know that the formation of cellular structures depends, at the same time, on the plasma proteins (eg. fibrinogen [5, 6]), on the local hematocrit, on the erythrocyte deformability, on the aggregation tendency and on the conditions of blood flow [7]. Erythrocyte aggregation results, from the interactions between deformable particles, red cells and from the center of a fluid carrier, the plasma. Every outside or inside cause susceptible of modifying these interactions will have an influence on aggregation and will govern the viscoelastic behavior or different *thixotropics* [3, 8]. In venous insufficiency, where the blood flow is low, when the shear rate and the shear stress are insufficient, the blood viscosity increases primarily because of the aggregation of red cells which, by an intercellular link of fibrinogen and of plasma globulins, arrange themselves in a network of aggregates which are more or less dissociable [2, 3, 5-7]. The measurement of microrheological parameters is essential for studies concerning pathological circumstances characterized by a hyperviscosity syndrome.

The increase of blood viscosity associated with an elevated incidence of venous thrombosis in vascular varicose vein patients tends to confirm for the clinician that hemorheological disturbances participate largely in the genesis of venous thrombosis [9, 10]. Thus, in these areas of stasis where blood flow is very low and where rheological abnormalities are major, the consequence can result in a decrease of oxygen pressure and in the accumulation of toxic cellular metabolites (ADP, free radicals). From a physiopathological point of view, the appearance and prolongation in time and space of an hyperviscosity syndrome, even local, entails rheological modifications : the capacity of the red blood cells to the carried by the axial current disappears, the aggregates are formed, these disturb the conditions of blood flow which may result in the cessation of flow, of lesions on the tissue by anoxia and finally in thrombosis [11, 12]. In veins, where the rate of blood flow is the lowest and where a stasis is frequent at the time of varicose veins, erythrocyte aggregation appears as the fundamental parameter in the comprehension of rheological abnormalities of blood. All the more, the aggregation is controlled by numerous factors such as shear rate, hematocrit, intrinsic properties of erythrocytes, fibrinogen and the chemical or physical properties of the environment. An excess of local aggregation or an increase of the threshold of disaggregation leads the appearance of pathological aggregates [13, 14], by the formation of inter-erythrocytary links of fibrinogen [7, 15, 16]. Hematocrit, fibrinogen level, plasma viscosity and increased aggregation index of red cells, in situations of circulation at low shear rate, diminish the transport of oxygen leading to a relative hypoxia. This, aggravated by a decrease in erythrocyte deformability, influences equally the exchange of transcapillary liquids. In fact, the preferential increase of post-capillary resistance which results in these disturbances, in relation to precapillary resistance, elevates capillary pressure to a transcapillary passage of liquid provoking hemoconcentration, tissular œdema, an acidosis and a liberation and accumulation of aggregates and toxic substances.

Material and methods

A double blind test against placebo, was carried out on 45 subjects : 20 control subjects, 25 patients – 13 receiving the *Ruscus* extract in doses of 2 pills per day, in 2 doses, and 12 receiving a placebo.

Population

The 20 control subjects had no venous insufficiency, and were without medical treatment, without oral contraceptives and within the 95 % range of the ideal weight, according to the International Committee for Standardization in Haematology [17]. All had a packed cell volume (PCV) and erythrocyte indices, mean cell volume (MCV) and mean cell hemoglobin concentration (Mc Hc) within the normal range.

The 25 subjects suffering from venous insufficiency were characterized by varicose vein of the lower limbs, non smokers, without metabolic disease, with no history of previous thrombosis disease, without medical treatment or oral contraception.

Microrheological parameters

The hematocrit was measured by microcentrifugation at 12 500 g for 5 minutes (1/1) ; plasma fibrinogen (g/l) was determined by using a thrombin clotting time technique [18]; plasma viscosity (mPa.s) was measured at 37°C by a KSPV4 capillary viscometer [19]; red cell deformability was evaluated by filtration measurements using an initial flow rate method as described by Hanss [20]. This method consists of the filtration of a diluted red cell suspension in buffer medium through nucleopore polycarbonate sieves with 5 µ diameter pores. The red cell aggregation phenomenon was quantified by the Sefam erythroaggregameter [21]. This device consists of an automatic Couette viscometer. The blood suspensions, placed in a narrow gap between two co-axial cylinders and lightened by a laser beam, are subjected to a high shear rate (600 s-1) leading to a complete disaggregation of red cells. The shear rate, which is suddenly stopped, allows the "rouleaux" formation. The changes in backscattered light through the blood suspensions are then recorded versus time. The final aggregation time, corresponding to the reciprocal of the slope of the plot and calculated between 40 sec and 60 sec is expressed in seconds and corresponds to the evaluations of the rates of " rouleaux" formation. In addition, the apparatus enables one to investigate the shear rate required for the disaggregation of red cell suspensions. This can be performed as follows: the blood sample is sequentially submitted to decreasing shear rates ranging from 600 s–1 to 7 s–1; each shear rate being followed by a lag-time of 5 sec. This leads to the plot of the reflected flux versus shear rate, illustrating a critical shear rate below which the reflected flux tends to decrease. This phenomenon indicates that the shear rate applied to the aggregates is not enough to allow the dispersion of red blood cell aggregates. From this shear rate, one can define [22, 23] the critical shear stress necessary to induce the dispersion of the red cell aggregates. The disaggregation shear rate is expressed in sec–1.

Another apparatus (Myrenne aggregameter AMM1) [24] has been also used in order to investigate the kinetic of erythrocyte aggregation. This technique allows the analysis of the optical changes of the blood (its increase in light transmission) in a transparent cone-plate-chamber. The measuring principle can be described as follows: the blood sample is first sheared at 600 s–1 and is then suddenly stopped or brought to a low shear rate of 3 s–1. The aggregate formation in both cases in accompanied by an increase in light transmission. From the plot of the transmitted light as a function of time, the area below the curve in the first 10 seconds subsequent to flow stop or reducing flow is calculated and is respectively called M1 and M2. These parameters are related to the extent of red cell aggregation and have been shown [24] to be fairly well correlated with the rate constant of the aggregation process. The value of M2 is higher than M1 because of the increased probability of the red cell interaction at a low shear rate which leads to a more accelerated aggregation rate than that of red cell aggregation at rest.

All the measurements have been made at the ambiant temperature of the laboratory (22+–2°C) in the hour after blood sampling with the exception of plasma viscosity (37°C) and of red cell aggregation by Sefam erythroaggregameter (37°C).

The blood samples were collected before and after 30 days of treatment by *Ruscus* extract or placebo, from the veins of the legs before and after 10 minutes of venous stasis with a hyperpressure of 10 mmHg controlled by plethysmography.

Statistical analysis

Differences in mean values between different parameters and different groups were assessed by the Student's t-test.

Results

Hematocrit (Table I)

Before treatment, the controls did not have a significant increase in the hematocrit value, regardless of the hemodynamic conditions (at rest and after stasis). By contrast, the patients had a significant increase of the hematocrit values after stasis. After treatment, we observed that the placebo group always had a significant increase of the hematocrit value, but the *Ruscus* extract group did not exhibit an increase of the hematocrit after stasis.

Fibrinogen (Table I)

Before treatment, the fibrinogen concentration of the two groups of patients is significantly higher than that of the control subjects. The venous stasis did not significantly increase the fibrinogen level in the veins of the legs of the control subjects (2.71+–0.23), but in the patient groups, the venous stasis was accompanied with an increase of fibrinogen level although the increase was not significant. After treatment for the two groups of patients, no modification in the fibrinogen concentration was observed, before and after stasis.

Plasma viscosity (Table I)

Before treatment and at rest, the plasma viscosity was increased significantly for the two groups of patients in comparison with the control subjects. After stasis, the plasma viscosity was not modified in the control group, but significantly increased in the patient groups. After treatment, before and after stasis, the placebo group showed no modification of the plasma viscosity values. The group of patients treated with *Ruscus* extract had a significant improvement of plasma viscosity after stasis in comparison to their plasma viscosity before treatment in the same hemodynamic conditions and in comparison to the placebo group (1.45+–0.02 versus 1.32+–0.02 $p<0.01$; 1.41+–0.02 versus 1.32+–0.02 $p<0.01$). Thus patients receiving *Ruscus* extract had plasma viscosity before and after stasis comparable to that to the controls, i.e. the stasis is not accompanied by an increase in plasma viscosity.

Table I. – Evolution of hematocrit, fibrinogen, plasma viscosity before and after venous stasis in control subjects and in two groups of patients suffering from venous insufficiency before and after treatment with *Ruscus* extract or placebo. Measurements on blood samples collected in veins of legs at rest and after controlled venous stasis. Results are expressed as mean + – SEM. *p<0.05, **p<0.01, ***p<0.001.

	Before Treatment		After Treatment	
	At rest	After stasis	At rest	After stasis
Hematocrit %				
Controls n=20	42.5±0.8	43.4±0.9		
Placebo n=12	40.4±0.9 —*— 43.8±0.8		41.4±0.7 —*— 44.5±1	
Ruscus extract n=13	41±0.7 —*— 43.9±1.4		41.2±0.8	42.4±1
Fibrinogen g/l				
Controls n=20	2.41±0.17	2.71±0.23		
Placebo n=12	*— 2.81±0.3	*— 3.31±0.4	2.81±0.2	3.1±0.17
Ruscus extract n=13	3.30±0.1	3.54±0.15	3.14±0.14	3.26±0.11
Plasma viscosity mPa.s				
Controls n=20	1.29±0.02	1.31±0.018		
Placebo n=12	1.34±0.02 —**— 1.42±0.03		1.35±0.02 —**— 1.41±0.02	
Ruscus extract n=13	1.33±0.02 —**— 1.45±0.02		1.30±0.01	1.32±0.02

Red cell deformability (Table II)

Before treatment and at rest, the red cell deformability index was identical in the control group and in the patients groups. After venous stasis, the red cell deformability index in the two patient groups was significantly higher than in control subjects. After treatment, the patients receiving placebo did not exhibit an appreciable modification and after stasis, the red blood deformability index was always significantly increased. The patients treated with *Ruscus* extract, before and after stasis, showed a normalization of this red cell parameter. The red cell deformability index in the patient group of *Ruscus* extract treatment was comparable to that of the control subjects.

Red cell aggregation-disaggregation (Table II)

High shear rate (600 s–1)

Before treatment, the red blood cell aggregation index, before stasis, was significantly higher in the two groups of patients than in the control group. Whereas the venous stasis did not modify this aggregation index in the control group, in the two patient groups, the venous stasis was accompanied by a significant increase in the aggregation index. After treatment, for the placebo group, the RBC aggregation index was not modified before and after venous stasis. By contrast, patients treated with *Ruscus* extract present a significant improvement of this index, especially after venous stasis, the patient group has a red blood cell aggregation index similar to that of the control subjects.

Low shear rate (3 s–1).

Before treatment for the two patient groups, the red blood cell aggregation indices were significantly increased in comparison to those of the control subjects. The venous stasis was also accompanied by an increase, which was not always significant. After treatment, patients receiving *Ruscus* extract had a significant improvement and decrease in the red blood cell aggregation regardless of the hemodynamic conditions (at rest, after stasis); whereas in the placebo group the values were unchanged. At low shear rate, the red blood cell aggregation index, at rest and after stasis, was similar to control in the patients treated with *Ruscus* extract.

Aggregation time (Table II)

Before treatment, at rest, patients with varicose veins had a significant decrease of the aggregation time in comparison with the control subjects. The venous stasis was accompanied by a significant acceleration of the red blood cell aggregation, whereas this was not seen in the control group. After treatment the red blood cell aggregation was not modified at rest and after venous stasis in the controls; by contrast, in the treated group, before and after stasis, the red blood cell aggregation time was improved significantly (21.75+–4.6 versus 27.8+–3.7 at rest) (17.2+–4.3 versus 25.7+–4.1 after stasis). The venous stasis unlike in the placebo group, was not accompanied by an acceleration of the red blood cell aggregation

Table II. – Evolution of red cell deformability index, kinetic indices of red cell aggregation, red cell aggregation time and red cell disaggregation shear rate before and after venous stasis in control subjects and in two groups of patients suffering from venous insufficiency before and after treatment with or placebo. Measurements on blood samples collected in veins of legs at rest and after controlled venous stasis. Results are expressed as mean ±SEM, *p<0.5, **p<0.02, ***p<0.01, ****p<0.001.

	Before treatment		After treatment	
	At rest	After stasis	At rest	After stasis
Red cell deformability				
Controls n=20	10.05±0.5	10.8±0.6		
Placebo n=12	10.6±0.5	12.4±0.4	10.1±0.6	12.2±0.7
Ruscus extract n=13	10.9±0.5	12.8±0.6	9.56±0.4	9.7±0.4
Red cell aggregation (after shear rate 600 s–1)				
Controls n=20	6.08±0.65	6.28±0.62		
Placebo n=12	8.92±0.67	11.2±0.7	9.07±0.58	12.3±0.6
Ruscus extract n=13	8.51±0.77	10.8±0.63	6.67±0.52	7.12±0.62
Red cell aggregation (at low shear rate 3 s–1)				
Controls n=20	8.44±0.7	9.4±0.82		
Placebo n=12	11.45±0.9	12.63±1.1	10.8±0.7	12.1±0.9
Ruscus extract n=13	11.88±1.1	13.47±1.04	9.49±0.6	10.53±0.8
Red cell aggregation time (sec)				
Controls n=20	32.5±7	30.2±4		
Placebo n=12	25.5±4	19.4±3.8	23.9±4.6	20.2±4.5
Ruscus extract n=13	21.75±4.6	17.2±4.3	27.8±3.7	25.7±4.1
Red cell disaggregation shear rate (sec–1)				
Controls n=20	51.34±5.5	62.6±7		
Placebo n=12	74.4±6	82.9±5	72.4±4.9	79.9±6
Ruscus extract n=13	74.04±5.2	83.4±5.5	65.8±5.2	70.3±5.3

Red cell disaggregation shear rate (Table II)

Before treatment, the patients had a significant increase of red blood cell disaggregation shear rate, at rest; the aggregates of red cell were barely dissociable. After venous stasis, these aggregates were less dissociable, and venous stasis was accompanied by a deleterious effect on the red blood cell aggregates. In control subjects, venous stasis was not accompanied by an increase of red blood cell disaggregation threshold. After treatment, in the placebo group, the red blood cell aggregates were barely dissociable, but in the *Ruscus* extract group, the red blood cell disaggregation shear rate was not disturbed by venous stasis and significantly improved (although not normalized).

Discussion

The viscosity of whole blood depends on the flow velocity or on the shear rates and on the shear stresses. In the post-capillary venules as well as in small veins, the first contribution to blood viscosity in the red cell aggregation-disaggregation phenomenon. The second factor controlling blood viscosity is the cellular concentration or hematocrit. The third factor is the plasma viscosity which depends on the plasma proteins (e.g. fibrinogen, albumin).

The lowest shear rates are found at the venous side of the circulation; this shear rate coincides with the red cell aggregation [8, 3, 25, 26]. If there is a dilatation of vessels (varicose veins), this shear rate can be decreased and become very low if not completely null. In the same time, proteins as albumin can pass through the venule or vein wall and lead to an hemoconcentration resulting in an increase of fibrinogen level and an increase of red blood cells. It is this foreseeable that the red cell-red cell or red cell-endothelial cell interactions will be influenced depending on the modifications of red blood cell properties and of the plasma proteins.

In the present study, the results show that patients with varicose veins of the legs have significant disturbances of the main hemorheological parameters of the blood viscosity, and that stasis on the varicose vein side aggravates these microrheological disturbances and thus blood viscosity.

Ruscus extract treatment is accompanied by an improvement of several microrheological factors of blood viscosity; in fact it seems that *Ruscus* extract treatment leads to :

— a significant decrease in hemoconcentration mainly under conditions of venous stasis (hematocrit, plasma viscosity); this could be explained by effects on resistance vessels and the permeability of capillaries, venules and veins, or by an effect on interstitiel conjunctive and vascular tissue by anti-edema effect.

— an improvement of red cell deformability, and inhibition of the deleterious effect of venous stasis.

— an improvement of the tendency of the red blood cells to hyperaggregate, especially at low shear rates and even after venous stasis.

Thus, the clinical activity of *Ruscus* extract probably is due to facilitating the return of blood, decreasing the hemoconcentration in stasis, and opposing the hyperaggregation tendency of red cells and the adhesiveness of these cells to the vessel wall.

Our result confirm previous studies done *in vitro* as well as earlier clinical studies [27, 28]. A therapeutic improvement of the microcirculation and of the hemorheological properties of blood appear to be of importance in the disturbances of venous circulation.

References

1. Lowe GDO. Blood rheology and venous thrombosis. Clinical Hemorheology. 1984 ; 4 : 571-588.
2. Chien S., Usami S, Dellenback RJ, *et al.* Blood viscosity : influence of erythrocyte aggregation. Science 1967; 157 : 829-831.
3. Chien S, Sung LA. Bases physicochimiques et implications cliniques de l'agrégation des globules rouges. Hémorhéologie et agrégation érythrocytaire. Ed. EM Inter Paris, 1986 ; 122-147.
4. Schmid Schonbein H, Gallasch G, Volger E, Microrheology and protein chemistry of pathological red cell aggregation (blood sludge) studied *in vitro*. Biorheology 1973 ; 10 : 213-227.
5. Meril EW, Gilliland ER, Lee TS, *et al.* Blood rheology : effects of fibrinogen deduced by addition. Circ Res 1966; 18 : 437-446.
6. Wells RE, Garowski TH, Cox PJ, *et al.* Influence of fibrinogen on flow properties of erythrocyte suspensions. Am J Physiol 1964; 207 : 1035-1040.
7. Brooks DE, Greig R, Jansen J. Mechanisms of erythrocyte aggregation Erythrocyte mechanics and blood flow. *In* : Cokelet GR, Meiselman HK, Brooks DE (Ed), New York, AR Lise Inc., 1980; 119-140.
8. Chien S. Biophysical behaviour of red cells in suspensions. The red blood cell, 2nd edition, edited by D. Mac N. Surgenor, Academic Press, New York, 1975, 2 : 1031.
9. Goldsmith HL. Blood flow and thrombosis. Throm Hemost. 1974; 32 : 35-48.
10. Goldsmith HL, Karino T. Mechanically induced thromboemboli. Quantitative cardiovascular studies, clinical and research applications of engineering principles. Edited by Hwang NHC, Gross DR, Patel DJ, Baltimore, University Park Press, 1979; 289-351.

11. Chien S. Blood rheology and its relation to flow resistance and transcapillary exchanges with special reference to shock. Adv Microcir 1969; 2 : 89.
12. Schmid Schonbein H. Critical closing pressure of yield shear stress as the cause of disturbed peripheral circulation. Acta Chir Scand 1976; 10 : sup. 465, 142.
13. Lerche D, Klaus H, Kunter H. Study of aggregation of human red blood cells. Stud Bioph 1976; 56 : 21.
14. Volger E, Schmid Shonbein H, Gosen J, et al. Microrheology and light transmission of blood. IV. The kinetics of artificial red cell aggregation induced by Dextran. Pflügers Arch 1975; 354 : 319.
15. Farhaeus R. The suspension stability of blood. Physiol Rev 1929; 9 : 241.
16. Chien S, Usami S, Dellenback RJ, et al. Shear dependent interaction of plasma proteins with erythrocytes in blood rheology. Am J Physiol. 1970; 219 : 143.
17. International Committee for Standardization in Haematology. Guidelines for measurement of blood viscosity and erythrocyte deformability. Clinical Hemorheology 1986; 6 : 439-453.
18. Caen J, Larrieu MJ, Samama M. L'hémostase : méthode d'exploration et diagnostic pratique. L'expension scientifique, Paris 1975.
19. Jung F, Roggenkamp HG, Schreider R, et al. Ein neues gerät zur quantifizierung der blutplasma-viskosität. Biomed Tech 1983; 28 : 249-252.
20. Hanss M. Erythrocyte filterability measurement by the initial flow rate method. Biorheology 1983; 20 : 199-211.
21. Donner M, Siadat M, Stoltz JF. Erythrocyte aggregation : approach by light scattering determination. Biorheology 1988; 25 : 367-375.
22. Othmane A, Bitbol M, Snabre P, et al. Red cell aggregation in insulin-dependent diabetics. Clinical Hemorheology 1989; 9 : 281-295.
23. Snabre P, Bitbol M, Mills P. Cell disaggregation behaviour in shear flow. Biophys J 1987; 51 : 795-807.
24. Schmid Schonbein H, Volger E, Teitel P, et al. New hemorheological technics for the routine laboratory. Clinical hemorheology 1982; 2 : 93-105.
25. Stoltz JF. L'agrégation érythrocytaire : aspects thérapeutiques. Hémorhéologie et agrégation érythrocytaire. Ed EM Inter Paris, 1986; 164-171.
26. Quemada D. Rheology of concentrated disperse system. A model for non newtonian shear viscosity in steady flows. Rheol Acta 1978; 17 : 632-642.
27. Kiesewetter H, Blume J, Scheffler P, et al. Efficacité clinique de Cyclo 3 Fort associé à la contention dans les insuffisances veineuses chroniques des membres inférieurs. Gazette Médicale 1987; tome 94 : 10, 2-7.
28. Kiesewetter H. In vitro testung der rheologischen Wirkkomponente des Ruscus-Präparates Phlebodril. Interner Bericht, 1984.

7

Effect of *Ruscus* extract* on the capillary filtration rate

G. Rudofsky

Angiology Clinic and Polyclinic, Essen University Hospital, Hufelandstraße 55, 4300 Essen 1, Germany

The causal chain consisting of insufficient venous valves, inadequate venous blood removal with venous hypervolaemia, a resultant insufficient drop in pressure, and a rise in pressure in the capillaries producing dilation of the capillaries ultimately leads to microcirculation disturbances due to the retardation of perfusion, increased filtration of liquid, and exsudation of protein into tissue, and thus to the formation of edemas [4].

As damaged venous valves cannot be restored and intact valves in dilated varicose veins are no longer capable of closing, attempts are made to compensate for the increased venous pressure by applying external pressure with dressings or compression stockings, to increase the tissue pressure and at the same time to reduce the elevated filtration rate using capillary-sealing drugs.

Ruscus extract and trimethylhesperidin chalcone [3] have been shown to act on the filtration rate in various animal experiments and clinical studies [1-5]. However, it has been demonstrated in experimental clinical studies that different filtration rates were measured, depending on the group concerned. Thus, the change in capillary permeability produced by *Ruscus* extract in

---

* Phlebodril®

healthy volunteers with a venous capacity of 4.8 ml/100ml tissue was about 0.3 ml/min, whereas in volunteers with a venous capacity of 3.5 ml/100 ml tissue a change of only 0.1 ml/min was found. It therefore seemed reasonable to assume that the filtration rate measurable by plethysmography may be influenced by various physical characteristics.

To check this hypothesis a meta-analysis was therefore made of three studies with similar designs, to investigate the effect of various factors such as age, sex, weight and height, and venous capacity on the filtration rate.

Material and methods

Baseline data

Each of the three studies was performed as a randomized double-blind crossover. In the first two studies healthy volunteers were investigated, receiving 450 mg *Ruscus* extract and 450 mg trimethylhesperidin chalcone (TMHC) as a single dose or 184 mg *Ruscus* extract together with 184 mg melilot extract applied topically. In the third study female patients with CVI stage I received 6g cream (96 mg *Ruscus* extract and 96 mg melilot extract) as a single dose.

Method

The action of the test substances on capillary permeability was determined in the three studies with the same apparatus (Gutmann Periquant), using the increase or decrease in tissue volume and venous occlusion plethysmography in a standard procedure [7]. The occlusion time was 10 min, with a occlusion pressure of 80 mm Hg. The rise in volume between the 5th and 10th minutes of congestion was taken to be the filtration rate.

Evaluation

The effect of the various physical characteristics, venous capacity, dosage form, and diagnosis (healthy - CVI) on the filtration rate was at first examined in a stepwise, multiple linear regression. In each case the values measured before administration of the drugs in the three studies were used as the reference level.

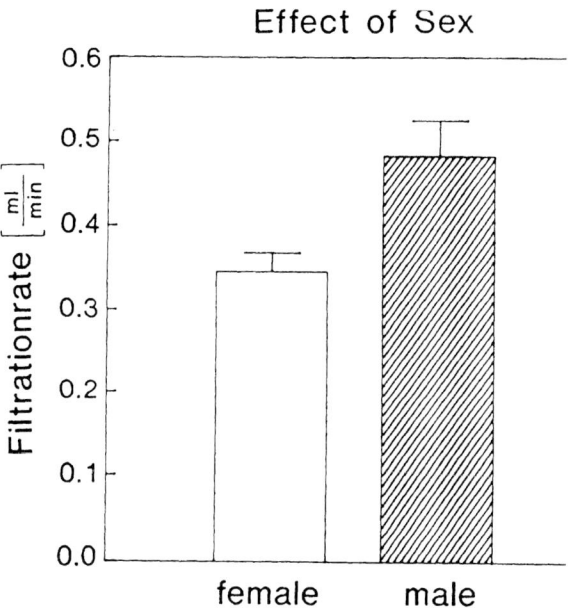

Figure 1. – Filtration rate of healthy volunteers; mean (x) and standard error (SE).

To demonstrate the action of the drugs, the factors identified as significant were then used as covariates in an analysis of variance (repeated measure design).

Results

The following correlations were identified in the regression calculation :
The filtration rate was not affected by age (p>0.10). Men have a filtration rate distinctly higher than women (p = 0.07) *(Figure 1)*. The filtration rate shows a significant drop with increasing Broca index (p = 0.005) *(Figure 2)*. As expected, in patients with CVI the filtration rate was clearly higher than in healthy volunteers (p = 0.033). The greatest correlation was found between the venous capacity and filtration rate (p < 0.001) *(Figure 3)*.

After adjusting the filtration rate for these factors, a highly significant treatment effect was found (p < 0.001). Within 2 h of the administration of *Ruscus* extract the filtration rate dropped by 0.17 ml/min *(Figure 4)*. This means

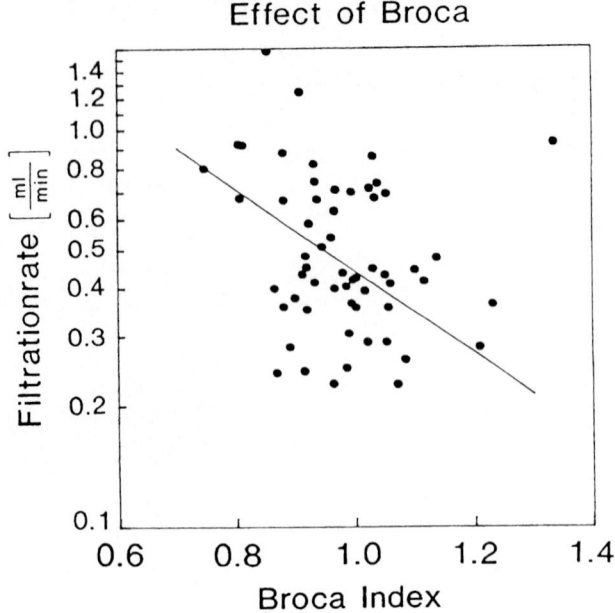

Figure 2. – Effect of Broca Index on filtration rate; n = 60.

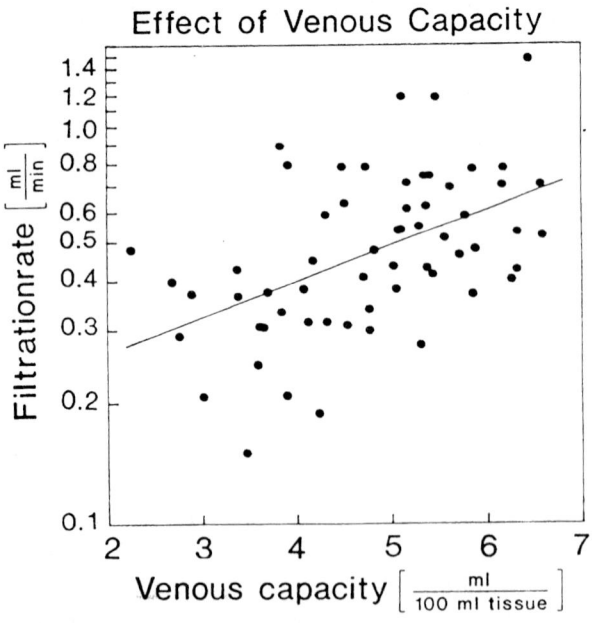

Figure 3. – Correlation between venous capacity and filtration rate; n = 60.

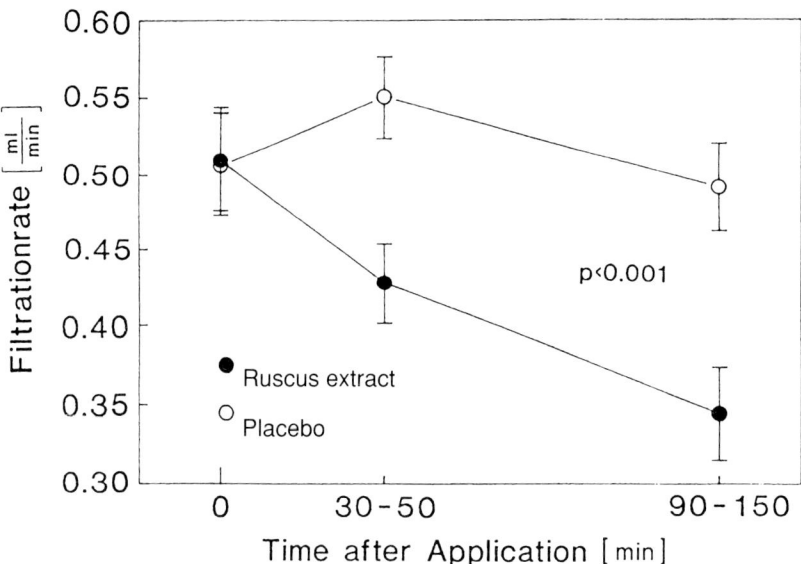

Figure 4. – Effect of treatment with *Ruscus* extract on filtration rate mean (x) and standard error (SE). The slopes of the curves differ significantly.

a decrease of 33 % referred to the baseline value of 0.51 ml/min. The duration of action was clearly longer than 2 h.

Discussion

The results show that *Ruscus* extract can exert a lasting effect on increased capillary permeability, one of the principal causes of microcirculation disturbance. The second characteristic of *Ruscus* extract, the tonic effect, has been demonstrated in animal experiments [12] and in clinical studies in healthy volunteers [3-5] and in patients [11]. Given the close connection between filtration rate and venous capacity, it could be assumed that a reduction in capillary filtration is achieved merely by increasing venous tone. This would mean that the same drug effect, i.e. the increase in venous tone, was measured by two different methods. However the highly significant effect of treatment on the capillary filtration rate after adjustment for the effect of venous capacity shows that the increase in venous tone and the reduction in capillary filtration are separate effects, but that both are produced by *Ruscus* extract in combination with TMHC or melilot extract.

This edema-protective effect is also supported by an improvement in lymph drainage. Thus, the lymphokinetic action of flavonoids and coumarin has been known for a long time [8, 9]. Animal studies demonstrate that the α-adrenergic action of *Ruscus* extract increased the motricity of the lymph vessels [10].

The interaction between capillary sealing and the increase in lymph flow should therefore produce a clear reduction in patients with venous edema congestion caused by chronic venous insufficiency, irrespective of its etiology. This has been demonstrated in a multicentre study with 141 patients [11].

References

1. Felix W, Nieberle J, Schmidt G. Protektive Wirkung von Trimethylhesperidinchalkon und *Ruscus aculeatus* genenüber Etacrynsäureödem am Hinterlauf der narkotisierten Katze. Phlebol Proktol 1983; 12 : 209-218.
2. Hönig I, Felix W. Effect on the permeability of isolated ear vein of the pig; a comparison between flavonoids and saponins. In : *Phlebologie' 89*. Davy A., Stemmer R. (eds), John Libbey Eurotext 680-682, London 1989.
3. Rudofsky G, Hirche H. Plethysmographische Untersuchungen eines Venentherapeutikums bei wärmebedingten hämodynamischen Veränderungen. Med Welt 1985; 36 : 145-149.
4. Rudofsky G. Venentonisierung und Kapillarabdichtung. Fort Med 107; (19) 430-434.
5. Rudofsky G. Transkutane Venentonisierung und Kapillarabdichtung bei gesunden Probanden. MMW 1989; 131 : (18) 362-365.
6. Schnitzer W, Klatt J, Baeker H, *et al.* Vergleich von szintigraphischen und plethysmographischen Messungen zur Bestimmung des kapillaren Filtrationskoeffizienten in der menschlichen Extremität. Basic Res Cardiol 1978; 73 : 77-84.
7. Rudofsky G, Esch P, Moser S, Ein Beitrag zur Standardisierung der Venenkapazitätsmessung. Act Chir 1984; 19 : 86-88.
8. Estler CJ. Zur Pharmakologie der Bioflavonoide. Fortschr Med 1971; 89 : 669-617.
9. Casley-Smith JR, Casley Smith Judith R. High protein œdemas and the benzopyrones. Lippincott Sydney, 1986.
10. Marcelon G, Pouget G, Tisné-Versailles J. Effect of *Ruscus* on the adrenoceptors of canine lymphatic thoracic duct. Phlebology 1988; 3 : (Suppl. 1) 109-112.
11. Rudofsky G, Diehm C, Gruß J, *et al.* Wirksamkeit einer Kombination venoaktiver Substanzen bei Patienten mit chronisch venöser Insuffizienz im Stadium I. In : *Therapie der Venener-krankungen*, Denck H., van Dongen R.J.A.M. (eds) 73-92, TM-Verlag, Hameln 1989.
12. Marcelon G, Vanhoutte PM. Venotonic effect of *Ruscus* under variable temperature conditions *in vitro*. Phlebology 1988; 3 : Suppl. 1, 51-54.

8

Microcirculatory responses to *Ruscus* extract in the hamster cheek pouch

E. Bouskela

Department of Physiology and Biophysics, University of Lund, Sölvegatan 19, S-223 62, Lund, Sweden

Introduction

Ruscus aculeatus is a very common plant, growing in all temperate regions of the world. The hydroalcoholic extract of its roots is used for the treatment of venous insufficiency, alone or in combination with other compounds [2, 3, 12]. The mechanisms of action proposed for *Ruscus* extract are (a) direct activation of postjunctional α1 and α2 adrenergic receptors and (b) displacement of stored norepinephrine from adrenergic nerve endings [8]. These activities have been demonstrated on veins and lymph vessels [7, 9, 10]. The present study was undertaken to determine the effects of *Ruscus* extract upon the microcirculation of the hamster cheek pouch (*in vivo* preparation). To our knowledge, there are no data available in the literature on the effects of this extract upon arterioles and venules, at the microcirculatory level. The routes used for administration of *Ruscus* extract, in this study, were oral, intravenous and topical. When topical application was studied, experiments were performed at different temperatures : 25 °C, 36.5°C and 40 °C.

Materials and Methods

For oral administration of *Ruscus* extract, twelve male hamsters, 7 to 10 weeks old, weight range from 75 to 120 g, were housed in individual cages and divided in two groups, R and W, 6 animals in each group. The animals received either 0.2 ml of *Ruscus* extract solution [(150 mg/kg), group R] or 0.2 ml of water (group W) daily, always in the morning, for 28 days. Every animal was observed at the microscope on the 29th day after the onset of the oral administration.

For intravenous and topical administration of *Ruscus* extract, experiments were also performed on male hamsters, 7 to 10 weeks old, weight range from 75 to 120 g.

Anesthesia was induced by an intraperitoneal injection of 0.1-0.2 ml of sodium pentobarbital (Mebumal vet., 60 mg/ml) and maintained with α-chloralose (100 mg/kg) administered intravenously. The femoral artery and vein were cannulated for pressure measurements, anesthetic and *Ruscus* extract injections. Throughout the surgery and subsequent experiment, the animal rested on a heating pad controlled by a rectal thermistor and body temperature was maintained at 36.5°C. A tracheal tube was inserted to facilitate spontaneous breathing. The hamster was placed on a stage containing a chamber with a silicon rubber ring surrounding a transillumination window. This chamber was preceded by another one which pre-heated the superfusion solution. Both chambers were mounted with Peltier elements for temperature control, allowing easy change and regulation of the superfusate's temperature. The cheek pouch was carefully everted with the aid of a moist cotton stick and the distal, non-muscular, part of it identified and pinned to a silicon ring [1, 13]. Dissection was performed under a stereomicroscope : a crescent-shaped incision was made in the top layer, the flap was pinned to the side and the areolar connective tissue removed to expose the bottom layer vasculature for microscopic observations. During the preparation and throughout the experiment, the cheek pouch was constantly superfused with a bicarbonate buffered saline solution (NaCl 131.9 mM ; KCl 4.7 mM ; $CaCl_2.2H_2O$ 2.0 mM; $MgSO_4.7H_2O$ 1.2 mM and $NaHCO_3$ 20.0 mM) at a rate of 4.6 ml/ min. This solution was continuously bubbled with 5 % CO_2 in N_2. This gas mixture was also continuously blowed through a perforated ring located on top of the transillumination window to assure that PO_2 in the superfusion solution bathing the pouch was maintained lower than 15 mmHg.

An intravital videomicroscope was used to observe the microcirculation and make microcirculatory measurement. The total magnification of the video image was 1000X. The TV monitor display was used to obtain arteriolar and venular diameter measurements by an image shearing monitor, IPM, model

907. During the whole experimental period, the diameter of arterioles and venules were recorded on videotape. In practice, we used videotape replay for final determination of vessel diameters, since greater attention could be given to this measurement than was possible during the conduct of the experiment. These measurements were recorded in a 6-channel stripchart record (Grass polygraph model RCS7C8).

For the oral administration part of the study, the experimental protocol consisted of sets of measurements performed on the same region in every animal. A venule with two side branches (collecting venules) and an arteriole with two side branches were measured in each preparation.

For the systemic IV administration part of the study, the experimental protocol consisted of sets of measurements performed every 10 min, exactly on the same site. During each set, data on vessel internal diameter as well as on arterial pressure were collected. The first 3 sets constituted the control period. After it, *Ruscus* extract, 5 mg/kg, was injected intravenously. The measurements started immediately after the injection and were performed every 10 min for 60 min.

For the topical administration part of the study, the experimental protocol consisted of sets of measurements performed exactly at the same site before and after different concentrations of *Ruscus* extract had been added to the superfusate. One to four arterioles and venules were studied in each animal. Six different concentrations of *Ruscus* extract were tested in every preparation : 5.10^{-3}, 10.10^{-3}, 50.10^{-3}, 100.10^{-3}, 500.10^{-3} and 1000.10^{-3} mg/ml. The animals were divided in three groups, depending on the temperature the cheek pouch was maintained during the experiment : Group I, 36.5°C ; Group II, 25.0°C and Group III, 40.0°C.

The results are expressed as either mean ± S.D., mean ± S.E.M. or ranges. Statistical significances were determined by the use of Student's t test and probabilities of less than 5 % ($P<0.05$) were considered significant.

Results

Oral administration

The animals were weighed once a week and there was no significant difference between the two groups *(Table I and Figure 1)*.

One animal of each group had problems during the surgical procedure and died.

E. Bouskela

Table I. – Body weight (g) of male hamsters receiving either *Ruscus* extract (group R) or water (group W)

Group	Day 0	Day 7	Day 14	Day 21	Day 28
R	90.0	90.0	95.5	93.4	95.9
R	100.0	100.0	115.3	113.5	114.5
R	95.0	100.0	108.1	110.0	112.6
R	100.0	100.0	113.2	114.0	113.7
R	85.0	85.0	87.1	85.2	88.5
R	85.0	90.0	94.1	97.4	93.7
W	90.0	95.0	106.8	107.2	107.4
W	95.0	95.0	103.6	106.2	108.7
W	100.0	100.0	105.7	107.0	108.2
W	80.0	80.0	82.8	84.7	87.0
W	90.0	90.0	97.1	100.2	102.5
W	80.0	85.0	94.1	94.7	92.9

Day 0 = onset of the oral administration

Table II. – Oral administration of *Ruscus* extract. Internal diameter (µm) of venules (V), venular side branches (SV), arterioles (A) and arteriolar side branches (SA).

Vessel type	Group R	Group W
V	42.82±3.28* (5)	60.76±6.80 (5)
SV	23.45±2.77 (10)	29.28±2.48 (10)
A	30.58±3.43* (5)	22.22±4.80 (5)
SA	14.77±0.86 (10)	13.78±1.25 (10)

Mean ± S.E.M.
(n)
* Significantly different from control (group W)

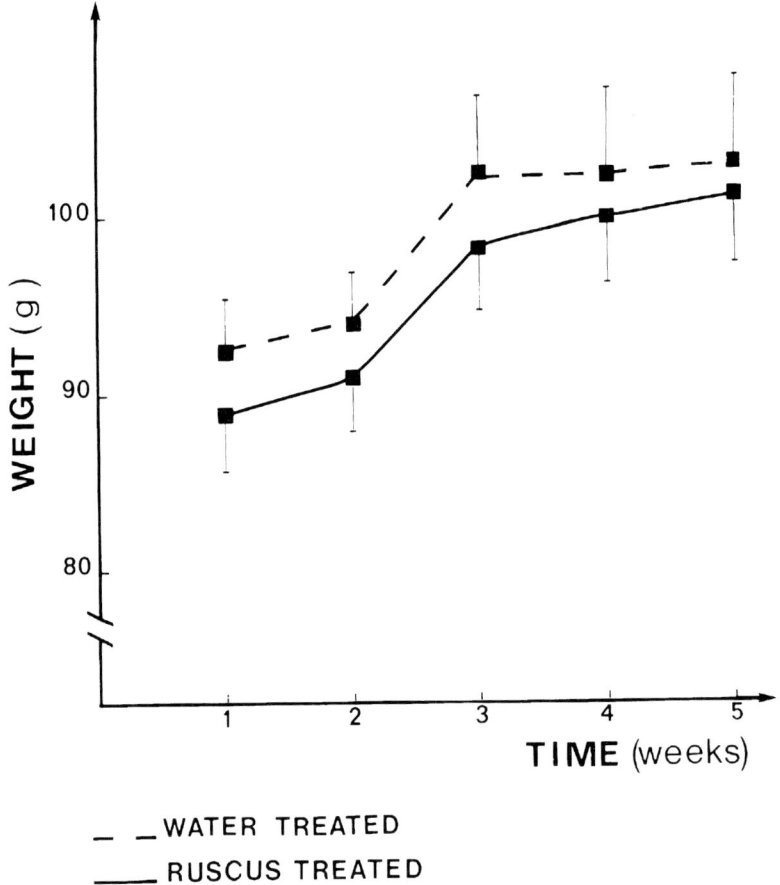

Figure 1. – Body weight of hamsters receiving either *Ruscus* extract or water (oral administration). Each point indicates mean ± S.E.M.

Mean arterial pressure was 95 ± 4 mmHg (mean ± S.E.M.) for the R group and 93 ± 7 mmHg for the W group.

The diameter of the studied vessels ranged from a) 35.0 to 85.4 µm for the venules; b) 10.9 to 42.8 µm for the venular side branches; c) 14.8 to 38.6 µm for the arterioles and d) 9.6 to 20.5 µm for the arteriolar side branches.

Oral administration of *Ruscus* extract (150 mg/kg during 28 days) elicited a 30 % constriction of the studied venules and a 37 % dilatation of the arterioles. The arteriolar and venular side branches were not affected *(Table II)*.

Systemic IV administration

Studies were performed on 7 male hamsters, weighing 97.6±6.1 g (mean ± S.E.M.). Arterioles, diameter range 10.0 to 35.0 µm and venules, diameter range 15.0 to 63.0 µm, were observed. *Table III* summarizes the results obtained.

Systemic intravenous administration of *Ruscus* extract, 5 mg/kg, provoked venular constriction and did not affect the arteriolar diameter in any considerable degree *(Table III and Figure 2)*. Mean arterial pressure was not affected by the intravenous injection of *Ruscus* extract in the dose used.

Topical administration

Studies were performed on 18 male hamsters, weighing 95.0±9.1 g (mean ± S.D.).

Arterioles, diameter range 11.7 to 74.9 µm and venules, diameter range 23.3 to 134.5 µm, were observed. *Tables IV, V and VI* show the results obtained at 36.5°C, 25.0°C and 40.0°C, respectively. The effects of topical application of different concentrations of *Ruscus* extract on arterioles and venules depended upon the temperature in which the hamster cheek pouch preparation was observed *(Figures 3 and 4)*. At 25.0°C, arterioles and venules dilated. At 36.5°C, arterioles either dilated for topical concentrations up to 50.10^{-3} mg/ml of *Ruscus* extract or remained unchanged when higher concentrations were applied, while the venules constricted. At 40.0°C, arterioles either did not change diameter for topical concentrations up to 10.10^{-3} mg/ml of the

Table III. – Intravenous administration (5 mg/kg) of *Ruscus* extract. Internal diameter of arterioles (A) and venules (V).

	After	10 min	20 min	30 min	40 min	50 min	60 min
V	89.82±2.92* (24)	92.99±1.61* (16)	92.27±1.57 (15)	93.93±2.41* (18)	90.66±5.05 (10)	90.16±3.13* (15)	94.34±2.66* (16)
A	100.30±2.14 (17)	96.42±1.81 (10)	98.94±3.03 (13)	100.52±3.64 (10)	102.13±3.05 (11)	98.74±3.79 (10)	95.30±3.35 (10)

To facilitate the comparison, the values are expressed as percentage of control dimensions. Mean ± S.E.M.
(n)
* Significantly different from control (P<0.05).

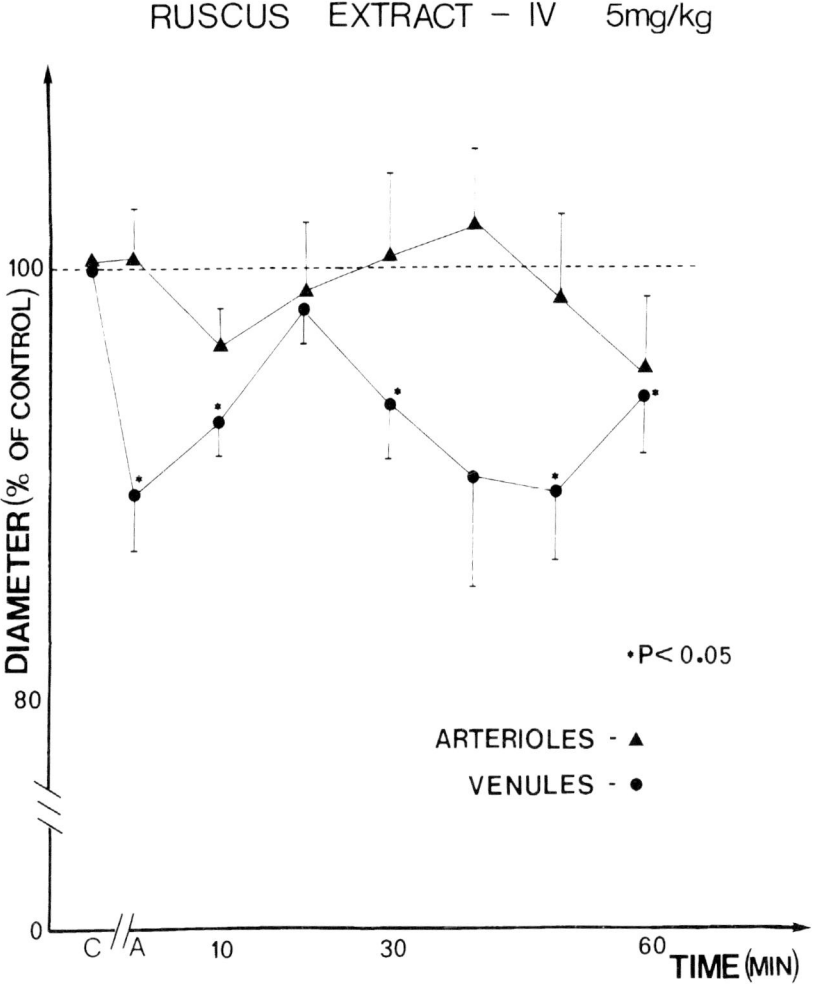

Figure 2. – Internal diameter changes of arterioles and venules after intravenous administration of *Ruscus* extract (5 mg/kg). To facilitate the comparison, the values are expressed as percentage of control dimensions. Each point indicates mean ± S.E.M.

extract or constricted when higher concentrations were applied, while the venules constricted.

Mean arterial pressure and the temperature of the animal were not affected by the experimental procedures.

Table IV. – Topical administration of *Ruscus* extract. Hamster cheek pouch microcirculation at 36.5°C

	Concentration of *Ruscus* extract (mg/ml)		
	5.10^{-3}	10.10^{-3}	50.10^{-3}
Arterioles	113.54±5.98 (8)	113.60±6.23 (8)	103.98±2.68 (8)
Venules	95.94±2.40 (13)	95.46±2.18 (13)	92.30±2.23* (19)
	100.10^{-3}	500.10^{-3}	1000.10^{-3}
Arterioles	100.32±3.36 (11)	102.77±3.87 (11)	102.66±4.96 (11)
Venules	92.28±2.01* (19)	88.85±1.31* (19)	88.64±2.48* (19)

To facilitate the comparison, the values are expressed as percentage of control dimensions.
Mean ± S.E.
(n)
* Significantly different from control

Table V. – Topical administration of *Ruscus* extract. Hamster cheek pouch microcirculation at 25.0°C

	Concentration of *Ruscus* extract (mg/ml)		
	5.10^{-3}	10.10^{-3}	50.10^{-3}
Arterioles	108.08±2.54* (11)	111.65±3.37* (11)	113.10±3.72* (11)
Venules	104.35±3.66 (22)	106.94±2.76*† (22)	105.47±3.42† (22)
	100.10^{-3}	500.10^{-3}	1000.10^{-3}
Arterioles	118.58±2.75*† (11)	118.03±2.94*† (11)	111.03±4.92* (11)
Venules	108.07±2.87*† (22)	106.73±2.82*† (22)	111.67±2.65*† (22)

To facilitate the comparison, the values are expressed as percentage of control dimensions.
Mean ± S.E.
(n)
* Significantly different from control ($P<0.05$)
† Significantly different from the 36.5°C value

Table VI. – Topical administration of *Ruscus* extract. Hamster cheek pouch microcirculation at 40.0°C.

	Concentration of *Ruscus* extract (mg/ml)		
	$5 \cdot 10^{-3}$	$10 \cdot 10^{-3}$	$50 \cdot 10^{-3}$
Arterioles	103.64±1.53 (12)	102.93±2.19 (12)	97.00±1.68† (12)
Venules	93.32±0.71* (20)	90.24±0.72*† (20)	85.50±1.28*† (20)
	$100 \cdot 10^{-3}$	$500 \cdot 10^{-3}$	$1000 \cdot 10^{-3}$
Arterioles	94.00±2.02* (12)	87.97±1.23*† (12)	84.32±0.97*† (12)
Venules	82.39±1.57*† (20)	77.73±1.86*† (20)	75.70±1.86*† (20)

To facilitate the comparison, the values are expressed as percentage of control dimension
Mean S.E.
(n)
* = significantly different from control (P<0.05)
† = significantly different from the 36.5°C value

Discussion

Several studies have demonstrated that *Ruscus* extract improves venous insufficiency. Rudofsky [11] reported a decrease of approximately 10 % in venous capacity 2h after oral administration of *Ruscus* extract in healthy volunteers.

Patients suffering from chronic venous insufficiency, treated with *Ruscus* extract, maintained a constant venous tone and improved venous emptying, unlike placebo patients [6]. In isolated canine saphenous veins, the extract of the roots of *Ruscus aculeatus* caused contractions [9]. Rubanyi et al. [10] showed that local warming augmented the venoconstriction evoked by *Ruscus* extract possibly because it facilitated the α1 adrenergic component of the venous smooth muscle response to the extract. Moderate cooling (from 37°C to 24°C) affects α-adrenergic contractile responses in canine cutaneous and deep veins differently [4]. By cooling, contractile responses to norepinephrine or sympathetic nerve stimulation are augmented in cutaneous veins

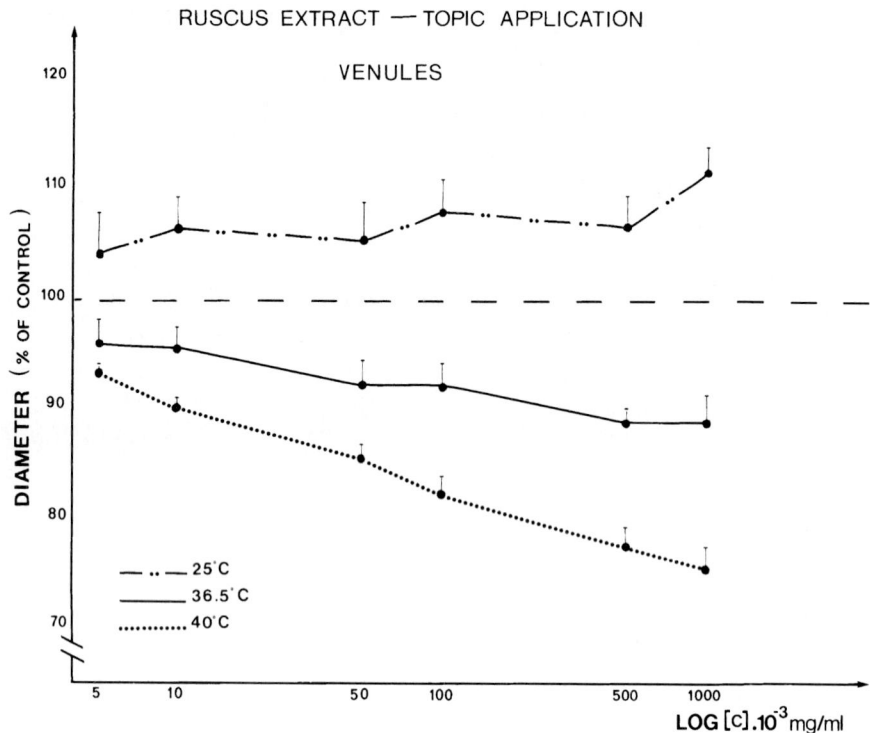

Figure 3. – Internal diameter changes of venules after topical application of different concentrations of *Ruscus* extract. Experiments were performed at 25.0°C, 36.5°C and 40.0°C. To facilitate the comparison, the values are expressed as percentage of control dimensions. Each point indicates mean ± S.E.M.

and depressed in the deep ones. In rings of saphenous veins, from control rabbits, *Ruscus* extract evoked concentration dependent contractions which were insensitive to prazosin and rauwolscine [5]. Cooling augmented these contractions and warming caused an increase in tone.

In our study, oral administration of *Ruscus* extract elicited a 30 % constriction of venules with internal diameter larger than 35 µm. The smaller venules were not affected. These findings could be explained by (a) lack of well defined smooth muscle layer and/or (b) lack of nerve endings in the smaller venules.

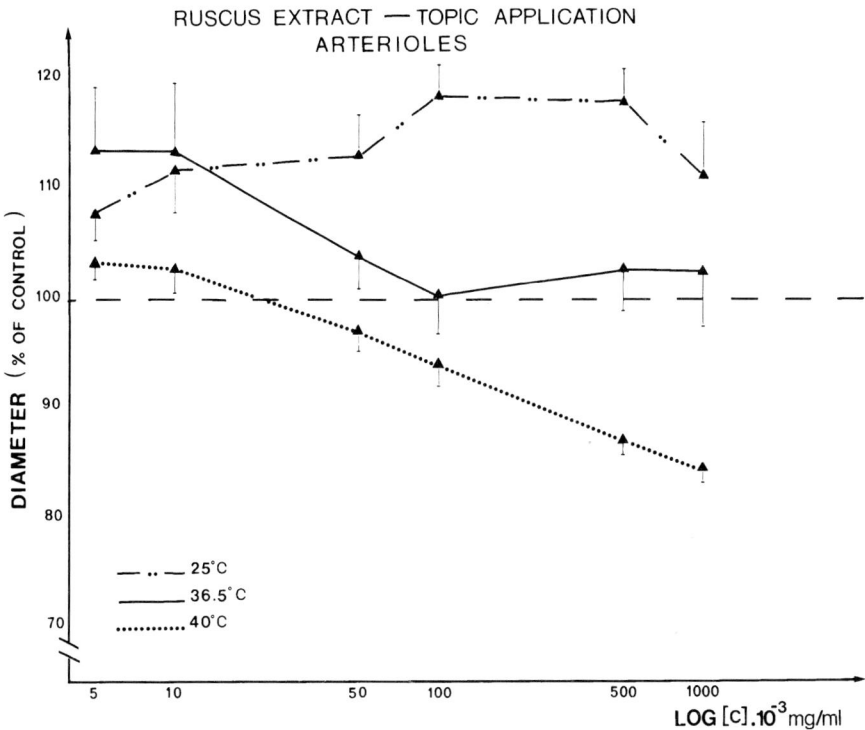

Figure 4. – Internal diameter changes of arterioles after topical application of different concentrations of *Ruscus* extract. Experiments were performed at 25.0°C, 36.5°C and 40.0°C. To facilitate the comparison, the values are expressed as percentage of control dimensions. Each point indicates mean ± S.E.M.

Systemic intravenous administration of *Ruscus* extract evoked venular constriction and did not affect the arteriolar diameter.

Topical application of *Ruscus* extract elicited concentration and temperature dependent responses in the studied vessels. At 25.0°C, arterioles and venules dilated; at 36.5°C, arterioles dilated or remained unchanged depending on the concentration used, while the venules constricted and at 40.0°C, arterioles remained unchanged or constricted depending on the concentration used while the venules constricted.

The observed differences between the responses of arterioles and venules after *Ruscus* extract administration could be explained by an augmented liberation of endothelium-derived relaxing factor on the arteriolar side (Miller *et al.*, this volume).

In conclusion, the effects of *Ruscus* extract observed *in vivo*, at microcirculatory level, are in agreement with the data previously reported in the literature on larger blood vessels and in patients with venous insufficiency.

Acknowledgements

The author wishes to thank Pierre Fabre Medicament for the generous supply of *Ruscus* extract. The skillful assistance of Ms. Fatima Z.G.A. Cyrino is also gratefully acknowledged.

References

1. Duling BR. The preparation and use of the hamster cheek pouch for studies of the microcirculation. Microvasc Res 1973; 5:423-429.
2. Elbaz C, Nebot F, Reinharez D. Insuffisance veineuse des membres inférieurs. Etude contrôlée de l'action du Cyclo 3. Phlébologie 1976; 29 (1):77-84.
3. Fayolle J. Cyclo 3: Indications thérapeutiques actuelles en phlébologie médicale. Cah Méd Lyonnais 1970; 46:1497-1498.
4. Flavahan NA, Vanhoutte PM Thermosensitivity of cutaneous and deep veins. Phlebology 1988; 3 (suppl. 1): 41-45.
5. Harker CT, Marcelon G, Vanhoutte PM. Temperature, oestrogens and contractions of venous smooth muscle of the rabbit. Phlebology 1988; 3 (suppl. 1):77-82.
6. Lozes A, Boccalon H. Double blind study of *Ruscus* extract: venous plethysmographic results in man. Inter Angio 1984; 3:99-102.
7. Marcelon G, Pouget G, Tisne-Versailles J. Effect of *Ruscus* on the adrenoceptors of the canine lymphatic thoracic duct. Phlebology 1988; 3 (suppl. 1):109-112.
8. Marcelon G, Vanhoutte PM. Mechanisms of action of *Ruscus* extract. Inter Angio 1984; 3:74-76.
9. Marcelon G, Verbeuren TJ, Lauressergues H, *et al.* Effect of *Ruscus aculeatus* on isolated canine cutaneous veins. Gen Pharmac 1983; 14:103-106.
10. Rubanyi G, Marcelon G, Vanhoutte PM. Effect of temperature on the responsiveness of cutaneous veins to the extract of *Ruscus aculeatus*. Gen Pharmac 1984; 15:431-434.
11. Rudofsky G. Plethysmographic studies of venous capacity and venous outflow and venotropic therapy. Inter Angio 1984; 3:95-98.
12. Sicard P. Resultats avec Cyclo 3 dans le traitement des ulcères variqueux. Phlébologie 1971; 1:117-121.
13. Svensjö E, Arfors KE, Arturson G. *et al.* The hamster cheek pouch preparation as a model for studies of macromolecular permeability of the microvasculaire. Uppsala J Med Sci 1978; 83:71-79.

Author Index

BOISSEAU, M.R.,	1
BONDOUX, G.,	57
BOULANGER, C.,	31
BOUSKELA, E.,	75
BRUCKNER, G.,	21
GROSET, M.,	41
HAJARINE, M.,	41
KHODABANDEHLOU, T.,	57
LAGARDE, M.,	41
LE DEVEHAT, C.,	57
LÜSCHER, Th. F.,	31
RUDOFSKY, G.,	69
SCHIMOKAWA, H.,	31
SCHINI, V.B.,	31
SVENSJÖ, E.,	47
VANHOUTTE, P.M.,	31
VIMEUX, M.,	57

LOUIS-JEAN
avenue d'Embrun, 05003 GAP cedex
Tél. : 92.53.17.00
Dépôt légal : 111 — Février 1992
Imprimé en France